Melissa Dingfi

The Psychology of Dental Care
Second Edition

DENTAL HANDBOOKS

Child Management in Dentistry (Second Edition)
G.Z. Wright, P.E. Starkey and D.E. Gardner

Complete Dentures
J.A. Hobkirk

Dental Care for Handicapped Patients
B. Hunter

Dental Treatment of the Elderly
J.F. Bates, D. Adams and G.D. Stafford

Endodontics in Clinical Practice (Third Edition)
F.J. Harty

Essentials of Dental Caries: The Disease and its Management
E.A.M. Kidd and S. Joyston-Bechal

General Anaesthesia and Sedation in Dentistry (Second Edition)
C.M. Hill and P.J. Morris

A Guide to Dental Radiography (Third Edition)
Rita A. Mason

**Killey and Kay's Outline of Oral Surgery
Part 1** (Second Edition)
G.R. Seward, M. Harris and D.A. McGowan

Local Anaesthesia in Dentistry (Third Edition)
G.L. Howe

An Outline of Oral Surgery Part 2
H.C. Killey, G.R. Seward and L.W. Kay

Outline of Periodontics (Second Edition)
J.D. Manson and B.M. Eley

Paediatric Operative Dentistry (Third Edition)
D.B. Kennedy

The Psychology of Dental Care (Second Edition)
G.G. Kent and A.S. Blinkhorn

DENTAL HANDBOOK

The Psychology of Dental Care
Second Edition

G.G. Kent PhD
Lecturer in Medical Psychology
Department of Psychiatry
Royal Hallamshire Hospital
Sheffield

A.S. Blinkhorn PhD, MSc, BDS
Reader in Dental Health and Honorary Consultant in Paediatric Dentistry
Department of Conservative Dentistry
Glasgow Dental Hospital and School
Glasgow

Wright

Wright
An imprint of Butterworth-Heinemann Ltd
Linacre House, Jordan Hill, Oxford OX2 8DP

 PART OF REED INTERNATIONAL BOOKS

OXFORD LONDON BOSTON
MUNICH NEW DELHI SINGAPORE SYDNEY
TOKYO TORONTO WELLINGTON

First published 1984
Second edition 1991

© Butterworth-Heinemann Ltd 1991
All rights reserved. No part of this publication
may be reproduced in any material form (including
photocopying or storing in any medium by electronic
means and whether or not transiently or incidentally
to some other use of this publication) without the
written permission of the copyright holder except in
accordance with the provisions of the Copyright,
Designs and Patents Act 1988 or under the terms of a
licence issued by the Copyright Licensing Agency Ltd,
90 Tottenham Court Road, London, England W1P 9HE.
Applications for the copyright holder's written permission
to reproduce any part of this publication should be addressed
to the publishers

British Library Cataloguing in Publication Data
Kent, G.G.
  The psychology of dental care. – 2nd ed.
  – (Dental handbooks)
  I. Title II. Blinkhorn, A.S. III. Series
  617.6

ISBN 0 7236 2339 2

Library of Congress Cataloguing in Publication Data
Kent, G., (Gerald)
  The psychology of dental care / G. Kent, A.S. Blinkhorn. — 2nd
ed.
    p. cm.
  Includes bibliographical references and index.
  ISBN 0 7236 2339 2.
  1. Dentistry--Psychological aspects. 2. Dentist and patient.
I. Blinkhorn, A. S. II. Title.
  [DNLM: 1. Dental Care—psychology. WU 29 K37p]
  RK53.K46 1991
  617.6'01—dc20   91-19233
  DNLM/DLC   CIP

Composition by Scribe Design, Gillingham, Kent
Printed and bound by Clays Ltd, St Ives plc

Contents

Foreword	vii
Preface	ix
Acknowledgements	xi

1 The social context of dental care — 1
   What is dental health? — 4
   Epidemiological studies of disease — 7
   Utilization of dental services — 12
   The dental profession — 17
   Summary — 24
   Practice implications — 24
   Suggested reading — 25
   References — 25

2 Prevention: The educational and behavioural viewpoints — 29
   The educational approach — 29
   The behavioural approach — 33
   Individual differences — 45
   Designing a preventive programme — 47
   Summary — 52
   Practice implications — 53
   Suggested reading — 53
   References — 53

3 The nature and causes of anxiety — 55
   The nature of anxiety — 55
   The causes of anxiety — 66
   Summary — 74
   Practice implications — 74
   References — 75

4 Alleviating anxiety — 77
   Modelling — 80
   Reducing uncertainty — 82
   Emotional support — 87
   Relaxation — 89

Cognitive approaches	92
Choosing between interventions	94
Summary	95
Practice implications	96
Suggested reading	96
References	96
5 Pain	99
The experience of pain	99
Measuring pain	104
Alleviating pain	109
Summary	118
Practice implications	119
Suggested reading	119
References	119
6 Special groups	122
Orthodontics	123
Temporomandibular joint disorders	125
The elderly patient	129
Patients with handicaps	130
Summary	132
Practice implications	132
Suggested reading	133
References	133
7 The dentist–patient relationship	135
Patients' perceptions of dentists	136
Communication	142
Teaching communication skills	149
Stress in dentistry	154
Summary	156
Practice implications	157
Suggested reading	157
References	158
Appendix 1 Some help for students	161
Studying	161
Anxiety during examinations	162
Conducting research projects	163
Further reading	164
Appendix 2 Case studies	165
Case study 1	165
Case study 2	166
Case study 3	166
Case study 4	167
Index	169

Foreword

It is a pleasure to write a foreword to the second edition of *The Psychology of Dental Care*. Since the first edition was published in 1984, there has been a growing awareness of the need for dentists and dental students to receive instruction and for experience of the application of the behavioural sciences in clinical dentistry.

In mid 1990, the General Dental Council published a report (General Dental Council (1990) *Guidance on the Teaching of Behavioural Sciences*. London: GDC) which concluded:

> The provision of dental care should not be seen in isolation from the psychological make-up and social background of the patient. Inclusion of the behavioural sciences in the undergraduate curriculum is intended to enable the student to move beyond the biological and mechanistic framework so as to view the patient as a complex sentient being with rights and expectations.

Among the main recommendations of that report were that the behavioural sciences should be taught throughout the course and beyond into vocational training and that dental students require courses in these subjects tailored to their special needs.

There is no doubt that the new edition of this book will be of great benefit to the teacher designing a new course and to the student desiring a deeper and broader understanding of this important subject. In this way it will help to raise standards of education and practice which will have consequential benefits to patients and I wish it every success.

Professor D.K. Mason

Preface

The oral health of the general population has improved substantially within the past decades. Overall, the incidence of caries and edentulousness has declined radically. As a result of this, many changes in dental practice and education will be needed within the professional lifetime of readers of this book. There will be a change from a restorative orientation to one in which greater attention will be given to high technological advances on the one hand, and to aspects of personal communication between dentists and patients on the other. This second edition has been written with the latter concerns in mind. Greater emphasis has been given to sociological aspects of dentistry and to the needs of patients who require particular forms of care, thereby helping the general dental practitioner to deal with nervous patients and improve communication skills.

This edition has some specific advice for students. We have attempted to draw out the implications of sociology and psychology for the practice of dentistry and also included Appendices which will be helpful for readers who are studying for examinations or are considering doing research in their own right.

G.G.K.
A.S.B.

Acknowledgements

For their assistance in commenting on earlier drafts of various chapters, we would like to thank Mary Dalgleish, Nick Fox, Peter Rothwell, Elizabeth Kay and Derek Attwood.

In addition to citations in the text, we would also like to thank the following for permission to reproduce material: Harcourt, Brace Jovanovich for Fier M.A. (1980) Hypnosis in dentistry: a case study. *Dental Survey* **56**, 12–13; Pergamon Press for Coe W.C. (1980) Expectations, hypnosis and suggestion in behavioural change. In *Helping People Change* (Kanfer F.H., Goldstein A.P., eds), London; the American Academy of Oral Medicine for Jackson E. (1975) Establishing rapport 1. Verbal interaction. *Journal of Oral Medicine* **30**, 105–10; and C.V. Mosby for Hirsch B., Levin B., Tiber N. (1973) Effects of dentist authoritarianism on patient evaluation of dentures. *J. Prosthet. Dent.* **30**, 745–8

Chapter 1

The social context of dental care

Many arguments could be made against the study of the behavioural sciences—which include psychology and sociology—in the dental curriculum. It could be said, for instance, that the teaching day is very crowded and students are asked to do far too much work already. Time taken in reading about behavioural science might be better spent in learning about anatomy and physiology, or practising restorative techniques.

Yet most dental schools now include the behavioural sciences as part of their curricula. Such professional bodies as the General Dental Council in the UK (1990) have argued strongly for their inclusion. The reason for this can be seen in any dentist's office. A practising dentist will meet a variety of patients on each working day whose dental health, or ill health, is due to the social context in which they live. On questioning, a dentist may find that one patient with severe toothache has suffered for many days before making an appointment. A child may continue to consume sugary snacks despite repeated warnings of what will happen to his or her teeth. An edentulous patient may return time and time again for further adjustments on a dental appliance even though by objective clinical criteria it is more than adequate. In all these instances, it is not the dentist's knowledge or skills about the technical side of dentistry which are most important, but rather the ability to understand why the patients are behaving in these ways. Dentistry cannot be practised in isolation from society, from other members of the dental team, or from the patient's family and social background. Just as a dental practitioner would not plan clinical care without a comprehensive treatment plan, it is unwise to predict human behaviour without some understanding of the behavioural sciences.

Table 1.1 illustrates some of the problems dentists encounter. General practitioners were asked to list 'three problems in managing patients which you find particularly troublesome'. The most frequent problem concerned the dentist–patient relationship. Sometimes this involved treatment planning (where a patient insisted on having the right to decide on the nature of treatment), while in other instances patients were rude or inconsiderate. The second most frequent difficulty was patient anxiety. Tense or agitated patients were not only difficult to treat but could disrupt scheduling or arouse uncomfortable feelings in the dentists themselves. Patients' failure to take adequate preventive care was another important difficulty. Although lack of information was seen to be an important cause of this for some dentists, others believed that many patients were unmotivated and unconcerned about their oral health. Some dentists stated that they found such patients frustrating and that their own motivation was declining (Kent, 1983).

Table 1.1 Problems cited as particularly troublesome by practising dentists in order of frequency

Rank order	
1	Dentist–patient relationship
2	Patient anxiety
3	Prevention
4	Dentists' personal feelings
5	Patients' unrealistic expectations
6	Practice management
7	Children's behaviour problems
8	Conflicts with parents over children's care
9	Patients' pain

From Kent (1983), with permission.

Aims of this book

This book has three main aims. The first is to explain some of the basic ideas in sociology and psychology as they relate to dentistry. This involves not only explaining the results of research, but also some of the difficulties in making sense of the results. This background is important because it is not possible to write a 'how to do it' manual which would be applicable to all patients and situations. Every patient is unique, but certain principles do apply. The skill is to recognize and use the principles when they would be helpful. Thus the second aim of the book is to provide the reader with the beginnings of a working knowledge of how the behavioural sciences can be applied in daily practice. A third and related aim is to assist dentists to make their occupation as rewarding and enjoyable as possible. Dentistry can be a stressful occupation, requiring a wide variety of abilities, but it is possible to see situations where patients complain or are unco-operative as challenging problems to be resolved rather than as sources of stress. It must be said that these are ambitious aims, and we may not always succeed, but we are confident that psychology and sociology offer much to assist dentists in their work.

Definitions of sociology and psychology

Sociology and psychology are complementary subjects. Just as an anatomist will concentrate on the structural aspects of the body and a physiologist will be more concerned with biological processes, one subject cannot be applied without an understanding of the other. Similarly, both sociological and psychological viewpoints are necessary for the understanding of how people behave. A sociologist is interested in the social and political organization of societies and how behaviour is influenced by the community in which a person lives. Such influences include large-scale factors as government policy towards funding the health services, allocation of resources between various specialties, and the beliefs held by people living in a culture about health and illness. In the USA, for instance, about 8% of the gross national product is spent on health care, while in the UK about half this amount is spent. As we will see, a person's socioeconomic status—whether he or she works in a highly paid professional job or a poorly paid manual one—is related to attendance patterns, dietary habits and the likelihood of caries development. A sociologist is interested in not only how these differences are related to dental care but also how they could be a reflection of the values and beliefs held by people in different communities.

Psychologists, on the other hand, are more concerned with individuals and their personal relationships. The social context is still vitally important, but there is more emphasis on individuals and their reactions to their environment. For example, a psychologist might be interested in whether some patients expect and experience more pain than others, or how edentulousness can affect self-esteem and willingness to engage in social activities. Some psychologists are interested in neurological mechanisms, but the main concern is with how these mechanisms affect behaviour. An individual may have a mental handicap due to a brain lesion, for example, but this becomes significant when it affects the ability to function in society.

Although there are these differences, there are also many similarities. Both psychologists and sociologists use some of the same terms and their shared aim is to understand why people behave as they do. Both are also concerned about social factors and how these have come to exert their influence on behaviour. The emphasis in this chapter is on how sociological factors influence dental care while later chapters concentrate more on psychological aspects.

Values and norms
Sociologists argue that the beliefs held by members of a society determine how they behave and react to others' behaviour. *Values* refer to collective beliefs. Some of the values of our society include a belief in democracy, the equality of individuals and the importance of professional health care. In a formal group such as an association of dentists there might be a collective belief in allowing all practitioners to offer private treatment irrespective of other contractual agreements. Such a value could be held alongside the collective belief that everyone should have access to dental care. On a more personal level, for example in the context of a family, there might be great value placed on scholastic endeavour, physical fitness or privacy. These values tend to be thought of in rather abstract terms and while they may be widely held in a society, some values may vary between sections of a society (e.g. dentists may place a greater value on oral health than others in the general population) or between families (e.g. one family may value regular atttendance for preventive care highly while another believes it to be less important).

Norms, on the other hand, are more concrete beliefs about behaviour. They reflect a set of beliefs about how people should behave in certain circumstances. A widely held social norm in western society concerns the view that professionals such as dentists should act impartially and according to a code of ethics. Among dentists there is a norm that 6-monthly check-ups are necessary for adults. A popularly held social norm among middle-class parents is that children should brush their teeth every morning and evening. If a person does not act in an acceptable way, punishments or sanctions may be applied in an attempt to correct behaviour. However, there is always a degree of latitude about these beliefs. Not all dentists agree about the importance of 6-monthly visits. Parents who have strict norms about brushing may allow their children to go to bed without brushing if they are very tired.

Socialization
Socialization is the term given to the process of learning values and norms. It is an ongoing and gradual process which continues throughout life. By the age of 3, for example, children know many of the basic norms and conventions practised in their culture, such as the 'correct' toys for boys and girls and the occupations which adult males and females typically enter. Children are very adept at picking up such rules and practise them during play. Conversations between adults and children often contain references to norms and values. The process of transmitting general cultural information is termed *primary* socialization. *Secondary* socialization concerns the values and knowledge base of a culture (Elkin and Handel, 1972). In western societies this is mainly transmitted in educational and work institutions. As will be seen later in this chapter, training in dental school involves socialization into the dental profession. This involves not only learning many technical skills but also learning the values and norms of the profession.

These sociological ideas of values, norms and socialization can often help in our understanding of behaviour in a society. Four major areas in which they will be met in this chapter are in problems of defining dental health, interpreting the results of epidemiological studies of disease, analysing the utilization of dental services, and examining professional issues.

What is dental health?

At first sight, this may appear to be a nonsensical question. A person could be said to be dentally healthy if he or she does not have any carious lesions or periodontal disease. But if this definition is used, then most people in the general population would be considered unhealthy. As discussed below, surveys have found that signs of clinically significant oral disease are very common and often untreated. Perhaps, then, a better definition would include some mention of a need for treatment. However, this answer also poses problems. It begs the questions of who makes a diagnosis and the decision to initiate treatment, what treatment is considered appropriate, and what is the ultimate aim of treatment? These judgements necessarily involve socially defined values and norms. In order to examine this basic issue of the definition of health, it is first necessary to make some distinctions between different kinds of ill health.

Impairment, disability and handicap

In an effort to broaden the scope of dental assessment from a purely biological to a social level of analysis, the World Health Organization (WHO, 1980) has suggested that a distinction be made between the objective pathology which a person may have and the disease's social and psychological effects. The WHO argues that the term 'impairment' could be used to refer to any physiological or anatomical loss or abnormality of structure or function. A broken leg, for example, is first of all an impairment. A fracture results in a 'disability' because it imposes some sort of limitation on activity, for example an inability to drive a car. Many individuals learn to live with their symptoms and come to an accommodation with the limitations imposed by disease. A third term is 'handicap'. The broken leg can be a handicap when it makes it difficult for an individual to fulfil his or her roles in a family or society. In this way two people could have a similar impairment but not share a handicap: a broken leg would be very handicapping for a travelling salesman who relies on driving to make a living, but much less so for a writer for whom mobility is less important. Similarly, a person with a severe reading problem due to a brain lesion may be handicapped and disabled in our highly technological society but not in a culture where most communication is verbal rather than written.

In dentistry, edentulousness provides a good example of these differences. The loss of teeth is an impairment, any resulting inability to eat certain foods is a disability, and an unwillingness to accept invitations out to dinner, lest some embarassment might ensue, is a handicap. Disabilities and handicaps do not reside solely within an individual but are always defined in terms of the person's interaction with the environment.

Disease and illness

A related distinction can be made between 'disease' and 'illness'. Like impairment, the term disease is used to refer to the organic pathology. Illness or 'illness behaviour' on the other hand, is subjective. It describes an individual's reaction to the disease. What people do in response to a disease depends on whether they notice any symptoms and how the symptoms are evaluated. Often, people will need to make a decision about whether a symptom is simply a transitory experience which will disappear of its own accord and so can be safely ignored, or whether it indicates a more serious condition. The first twinges of a toothache might be dismissed, being seen simply as a result of having a hot drink. Many people believe that it is natural for gums to bleed during brushing (Craft and Croucher, 1980) rather than being a sign of disease. As a result, no action is taken to seek a remedy.

Measuring dental health

Thus it is possible to measure dental health in several ways. When relying on clinical criteria several indices can be used, such as the decayed/missing/filled teeth (DMFT) score, or indices of plaque and gingivitis. The clinical signs of temporomandibular joint disorders (TMJD) include locking of the joint, sounds during movement, and pain on muscle palpitation. These measures may seem straightforward and objective, but in fact there can often be problems in assessment. The DMFT score is problematic. It is really a measure of dental history, rather than current dental health. Teeth may be missing because of planned extractions due to overcrowding, never erupted or perhaps the patient had an accident. The reliability of a measure is ascertained by asking at least two clinicians to examine patients independently. If both report the same results (i.e. if they agree that a sign is either absent or present), then their measures would be considered reliable. It is often assumed that all dentists would agree and come to the same conclusions when examining patients, but when this assumption has been put to the test some disconcerting results have arisen. For example Smith (1977) asked two dentists to examine patients for signs of TMJD. Smith found that there was total disagreement for 10% of the sample. For all the remaining patients, each dentist recorded many signs and symptoms not noted by the other.

As well as problems with interpretation and reliability, it has also been argued that such assessments are too narrowly based, giving insufficient attention to social consequences. That is, they concentrate on impairment while neglecting disability and handicap (Locker, 1988; Reisine, 1988). *Sociodental* indicators assess how disease affects individuals' lives. Here there is less concern with clinical criteria and more with how a condition affects an individual's self-esteem or ability to perform normal social activities. The effects of dental disease are widespread: Cushing et al. (1986) found that 26% of adults had experienced dental pain, 20% had difficulty in eating and 15% problems in communication during the previous year. Such discomfort can lead to high levels of disability or handicap for a patient. It is clear that some oral conditions, such as a disfiguring facial cleft, can have long-lasting and severe consequences on social and sexual relationships (Peter and Chinsky, 1974). So, too, can edentulousness. Several studies have shown that the wearing of dentures is associated with a variety of difficulties. These include not only disabling problems such as an inability to chew certain foods but also a greater likelihood of mandibular dysfunctions such as headaches (Carlsson, 1976; Magnusson, 1980) and social problems such as refusing invitations to other people's homes and avoidance of speaking (Blomberg and Linquist, 1983). Some scales, such as the Sickness Impact Profile (Bergner and Bobbitt, 1981) are designed to measure the effects of health difficulties on physical abilities (e.g. mobility, sleeping) and social roles (e.g. working relationships, recreation and communication).

The issue of how to measure dental health becomes very interesting when comparisons between clinical and functional criteria are made. Often the effects of a condition cannot be predicted by a knowledge of the severity of the impairment. This is shown most clearly by the research on denture patients. Attempts have been made in several studies to relate clinical assessments of denture quality on such criteria as retention, fit, stability and bite force to patients' satisfaction with their appliances, but these have been largely unsuccessful. For example, Heyink et al. (1986) found only weak associations between dentists' and patients' appraisals of dentures. For the patients, denture quality depended on how well they could function in practical everyday terms. Similarly, Haraldson et al. (1979) compared the bite force of patients who were satisfied or dissatisfied with their dentures. No difference could be found. Although such studies indicate that extremely poor-quality appliances are associated with the most dissatisfaction, the relationship is not a close one.

Such studies show that the values of dentists may not correspond to those of lay people. It is not simply a question of which group holds the 'right' or 'correct' beliefs. Rather, that the values may be different and that such differences have many implications for the practice of dentistry. For example, a dentist who is working from only a clinical set of values about the importance of disease will miss the role of the patient's point of view. A treatment plan, though clinically correct, may not be feasible because it is inconsistent with a patient's priorities and difficulties. As a result, the dentist and the patient may have different beliefs about what the treatment should entail.

Epidemiological studies of disease

The epidemiological approach to health care research provides one way of identifying factors associated with disease. An epidemiologist attempts to discover the rates of disease in various groups of people and then tries to relate this to factors in their lifestyle or environment. The studies conducted in the 1950s which found a link between lung cancer and cigarette smoking were based on this kind of work. Epidemiologists have drawn our attention to the influence of many aspects of people's lives, including age, income, and type of housing.

One of the central factors is social class. This concept has developed since the industrial revolution when jobs became more differentiated than in farming-based communities (Abercrombie and Warde, 1988). The division of labour led to the development of classifications based on occupation, such as the Registrar General's classification shown in Table 1.2.

Table 1.2 Registrar General's social class classification

Social class	Description	Examples
I	Professional	Doctor, dentist, lawyer
II	Intermediate	Manager, school teacher, nurse
IIINM	Skilled non-manual	Secretary, clerical worker, dental technician
IIIM	Skilled manual	Bus driver, carpenter
IV	Partly skilled	Postman, agricultural worker
V	Unskilled	Cleaner, labourer

Adapted from OPCS (1980) with permission.

8 The Psychology of Dental Care

In this classification all jobs are placed into one of six categories, each being assigned a social class. Social class I, for example, includes accountants, dentists, doctors and lawyers.

Edentulousness, age and social class

If an epidemiologist were interested in a possible relationship between social class or age and dental health, the information could be collected in several ways. One possibility is to consult dental records of patients living in two contrasting areas of a city, to ensure that all classes are represented, over a particular period of time. This would give an indication of the number of new cases seen by the dentist. The measures of dental health could include a DMFT score, the rate of edentulousness, or an index of periodontal disease.

This would provide an indication of the rate at which patients utilize the dental services for particular conditions, but it would not provide an estimate of the prevalence of a problem since not everyone who has a disease will seek professional care. In order to gauge prevalence, it is necessary to take a survey of the general population. The sample to be examined could be selected randomly or the researchers could decide beforehand to approach people from particular social groupings and ages. In the case of a project attempting to relate oral health with social class, people could be asked about their occupations and then assigned to groups. This is the method used in one survey conducted in the UK. The occupants of 10000 private households were interviewed in their own homes and asked about a variety of topics such as education, housing and income as part of a national census. A summary of the results relating to the rates of edentulousness is shown in Table 1.3; differences are related to age and social class.

Table 1.3 Percentage of adults with no natural teeth by age and socioeconomic group

Age (years)	Professional	Managers	Intermediate non-manual	Junior non-manual	Skilled manual	Semi-skilled manual	Unskilled manual
16–24	Nil	Nil	Nil	–	–	Nil	1
25–34	Nil	2	1	1	2	3	5
35–44	2	4	7	4	12	14	23
45–54	6	11	15	16	28	35	38
55–64	15	28	26	36	48	58	59
65–74	28	45	42	60	74	77	75
75 and over		73	74	77	84	89	88
All ages	8	19	16	20	28	36	44

Adapted from OPCS (1986).

Although the table is rather complicated, it indicates two main things. First, it shows that the rate of edentulousness varies across social groups. The prevalence of edentulousness is higher in households where the husband's occupation falls to the lower end of range of social classes. For example, in the age range 55–64, only 15% of the respondents from the professional level were edentulous, but this increased to 26% at the intermediate non-manual level and to 58% in households where the adult male was employed in an unskilled manual job. Second, Table 1.3 indicates that edentulousness is associated with age. There is a consistent increase in total tooth loss in all social groupings with increasing age.

One attraction of epidemiological studies is that if the same questions are asked at different times, changes in the prevalence of disease can be monitored. Table 1.4 illustrates another set of results from the same survey—a comparison of rates of edentulousness in 1968, 1978 and 1983. In all age groupings the prevalence of edentulousness was lower in 1983 than in earlier surveys.

Table 1.4 Trends in total tooth loss over time: percentage of adults with no natural teeth by age

Age (years)	1968	1978	1983
16–24	1	–	–
25–34	7	3	2
35–44	22	12	7
45–54	41	29	22
55–64	64	48	41
65–74	79	74	64
75 and over	88	87	81
All ages	37	29	25

Adapted from OPCS (1986).

Some difficulties in epidemiological research
While these results are very informative, there are some problems with this study. One problem is in the classification of social class, which was determined by the occupation alone. The most recent classification of occupations (OPCS, 1990) provides a very detailed classification system, but it is still a rather crude measure of socioeconomic status. It is helpful to take other factors such as income, housing and educational level into account when making a classification of socioeconomic status. One such indicator was devised by Jarman (1984). When surveying the prevalence of disease in different areas, he not only assessed occupation but also the number of elderly people living alone, children under 5, one-parent families, levels of unemployment and overcrowding. By taking this broader view it was possible to delineate areas more accurately in terms of social background and deprivation.

Perhaps the simplest indicator of whether a family has much disposable income is car ownership. The resources required to buy and run a car will be beyond people living at or below subsistence level. Car ownership also gives a family the gift of mobility. Using public transport may mean that a visit to a clinic is too difficult and it is not possible to shop at stores for fresh fruit and vegetables.

A second problem of the survey is that it relied on respondents' self-reports of their health and behaviour. There is evidence that self-reported data in this area need to be treated with considerable caution. Another question asked in this survey concerned the regularity of attendance at the dentist's. For dentate adults, 48% claimed that they attended for regular check-ups, 13% that they attended for the occasional check-up, and 40% only when they were experiencing some trouble with their teeth. But Eddie (1984) put such claims to the test by consulting the patients' dental records. Of a sample of people who claimed regular attendance, only 31% had actually done so in the previous 5 years, 53% had attended infrequently, and 16% not at all. Perhaps the people in the OPCS survey were replying according to their beliefs about how they should behave, rather than on the basis of their actual behaviour.

The decline of caries

Physical examinations are necessary when an epidemiologist seeks to estimate the prevalence of disease, such as carious lesions and periodontal problems. Studies in this area have indicated a steep decline in the incidence (or the number of new cases) of caries, especially in children and young adults and particularly in children from higher socioeconomic groupings. The estimate of the decline is substantial—by 30% to 50% over the past two decades (Burt, 1985). Burt (1978) cites a study from Norway on children between 6 and 17 years of age who received treatment from the school dental service. In 1966, 8 children per 100 examined required an extraction due to severe caries, but this had declined to 0.7 children per 100 in 1976. Similarly, 617.9 restorations were given per 100 children in 1966, but only 340.9 in 1976. These and many other results indicate that the level of caries in children is declining rapidly.

Explanations for patterns in disease

Sociologists are not content simply to describe patterns of disease. They are also interested in studying possible explanations for any differences. One general conclusion from their work is that many factors contribute to patterns of health and disease.

Social class differences

There are a number of possible explanations for the consistent finding of higher levels of disease in people from lower socioeconomic groups. One factor concerns the cost of professional dental care. People from poorer families are less able to afford regular visits to a dentist. But here the results are equivocal. Although irregular attenders often cite cost as an important barrier to care, this is not necessarily the only factor. For example, Kegeles (1963) studied the attendance patterns of the employees of a company which provided free dental services. Although 90% of the employees in supervisory positions consulted the dentist for preventive care, only 51% of those in non-supervisory positions did so, even though income was not relevant.

Another possible explanation for the relationship between health and socioeconomic level involves the values and norms held by different groups in society. Several writers have suggested that, as a generalization, middle- and upper-class patients tend to be more future-oriented and so more likely to take preventive actions. In a study on adolescents with rampant caries, Blinkhorn (1989) found that the majority of the adolescents came from a working-class background and tended to snack throughout the day on sugary foods. Cooked meals were seldom eaten, except for hamburgers and other fast foods. Attwood et al. (1990) have suggested that class differences in dental health are influenced by the following factors:

1. Children from affluent areas are more likely to use fluoride toothpaste.
2. The intake of refined carbohydrate is lower in the upper socioeconomic groups.
3. The parents from upper social class groups are more interested in oral health and seek advice and routine screening from a dentist more frequently.

Once such patterns have developed, it seems that they tend to persist over generations through the process of socialization. Parents' dietary and preventive practices are the best predictors of children's behaviour (Metz and Richards, 1967).

There is also the supply of dentists to consider. Middle- and upper-class areas of cities tend to be better served by dentists, so it is easier for people having professional and skilled occupations to visit a dentist (O'Mullane and Robinson, 1977).

It seems that all of the above factors can contribute to socioeconomic differences in oral health. Often the factors are found in combination (i.e. low income, cariogenic dietary habits and reduced access to dentists) and are all part of general social deprivation. In the UK, a Royal Commission on inequalities in health (Townsend and Davidson, 1982) highlighted the evidence of the failure of successive governments to overcome inequalities in health care provision. The main conclusions were:

1. Britain's health service does not work for people of lower socioeconomic levels.
2. The lower the socioeconomic level, the more ill health
3. Ill health is not just a result of failings in the health service but is linked to inequalities in income, education, housing and working conditions which affect people throughout their lives.

Caries decline
Against this background of inequality of health, however, lies the general reduction of caries in the general population. Although this is related to socioeconomic status (the decline of caries is greater in the higher socioeconomic groups), the sheer size of the caries decline is difficult to explain. Burt (1985) suggests three possibilities. One is that the count of *Streptococcus mutans* bacteria, the principal pathogen in caries development, is declining in the population. This could be due to the increased use of antibiotics for the control of other infections in children. A decline in *S. mutans* could be a happy side-effect of the control of other

bacteria. Another possibility is that there has been a decline in sucrose consumption. Although sugar consumption overall has not changed appreciably, high fructose corn sugar (HFCS) is being increasingly used in manufactured foods. Perhaps this is less cariogenic than sucrose. A third possibility is the increased use of fluoride, both in water supplies and in commercial toothpastes. This has undoubtedly been important and can in itself account for most of the decline. Improvements in housing and sanitation have had a huge impact on mortality and morbidity, radically improving general health (McKeown, 1979). It seems likely that the increased availability of fluoride has had a comparable effect on dental health.

Ethnic variations
Many of the early investigations of the cultural differences in response to symptoms were undertaken in the USA on immigrant groups (Opler and Singer, 1956). Gift (1985) reviewed the American literature on race and ethnicity in relation to the use of dental services and concluded that a larger proportion of whites than non-whites made use of them. However) income level was of over-riding importance and Moosbrucker and Jong (1969) concluded that there were no significant differences in dental visiting between individuals of different races with similar income levels. In the UK the dental health of ethnic communities does not reveal a consistent pattern. Williams (1984) reported higher caries levels in young Asian children. A more recent study found oral hygiene practices amongst young Asians were different from Caucasian children of a similar age (Williams and Fairpo, 1988), and there are marked differences in dental visiting patterns amongst Bangladeshi and white children. Only 3% of the latter had never visited a dentist compared with 30% of the Bangladeshi children (Laher, 1990). Such patterns could be due to many factors. The higher caries rates may be due to dietary or weaning differences between ethnic and indigenous people, but they may also be due to a move from a culture in which little sugar is consumed to the West's sugar-laden culture. That is, a family's oral health habits may have been 'good' when they lived in their original country but not suitable for Europe or North America.

Although these differences are marked, cultural variation can be given too much emphasis because in any single society patterns of disease and health care will vary quite dramatically between social groups. Many of the problems associated with minority status are in fact closely related to deprivation (Beal, 1990). Findings of cultural differences must be treated with caution as immigrant status and the stress of adapting to a new culture are important influences. Thus, when people seek health care or cope with symptoms in some other way they may be influenced not only by cultural background but also by their new social environment (Hochstein et al., 1968; Douglass and Cole, 1979).

Utilization of dental services

Sociologists have been interested for many years in the problem of why and when an individual decides to seek medical or dental care. Initially it was assumed that there would be a close correspondence between clinical signs of disease and the decision to consult a dentist. However, this has proven not to be the case and it seems that the processes that are involved in becoming a patient are quite complex. The British Adult Dental Health survey undertaken in 1968 (Gray et al., 1970) found that half the sample of respondents went to the dentist only when they had trouble with their teeth. By the time of the 1978 study (Todd and Walker, 1980), this proportion had dropped to 40%. In order to understand why the uptake of dental services is lower than one would expect it is helpful to consider the distinction between the *need* and the *demand* for care.

Demand versus need

Many studies have shown that a high proportion of people in the general population are in need of help from the dental services yet do not seek it out. Locker and Slade (1988) found that almost half of a sample contacted by telephone reported one or more symptoms of TMJD, but only 2.8% were receiving or had ever received any treatment. When a subsample was subsequently examined clinically, 88% showed one or more of nine signs of TMJ disorder: 26% had one sign, 19% had two, and 32% had three or more. Elderly people have been found to be in the greatest need of treatment on clinical criteria. Although it is a mistake to believe that all elderly people are in need of care (see Chapter 6), Smith and Sheiham (1979) found a remarkably high degree of disease and disability in people over the age of 65. About one-third of the sample said they were in pain, sometimes sufficiently severe to keep them awake at night. Twenty-five per cent of the full dentures examined were damaged and only 10% of maxillary and mandibular appliances were considered satisfactory by the dental examiners. A quarter of the appliances had been worn for over 20 years. Overall, 78% were considered to need some form of dental treatment (Smith and Sheiham, 1980). However such difficulties were infrequently translated into visits to the dentist. Only 19% of those assessed as needing treatment had tried to obtain it. Even among those who complained of pain the demand was low: 14% of those who were experiencing pain had seen a doctor or dentist about it.

Such differences between what clinicians believe is appropriate for people and the demand for their services can be found for all other dental conditions. Although there are some instances in which patients may make demands when the dentist believes treatment is not needed on clinical criteria, it is more usual for dentists to see only a small proportion— the tip of the iceberg—of the total number of people who are actually in ill health (Hannay, 1988).

Reasons for low demand

Many types of explanations for this discrepancy between need and demand have been put forward. Health professionals believe that the maintenance of 'good health' should be a priority for most people, but practising clinicians are well aware that individuals fail to arrive for appointments and live with painful symptoms (Blinkhorn et al., 1983).

Good health is only one part of a person's life and it may be less important than other more pressing problems. An individual will weigh up the potential costs of a health-oriented behaviour and then assess the potential benefits of seeking care (Woolgrove et al., 1987). Clearly this will not be an academic exercise in cost/benefit analysis, but a pot pourri of perceived barriers to seeking care, the importance attached to a specific health area and how friends and relatives view the symptoms. Thus, while need is defined by the values of health professionals, demand is a consequence of the valuation of health care by the consumers—the patients.

Barriers to dental care
Access to dental services can be restricted due to financial, political and emotional barriers, or to a combination of these. Low income can result in several disadvantages. Not only may a family who are struggling financially have difficulty in paying fees, but also in finding the money for bus fares or paying a child-minder when they visit. Someone who is self-employed might have to forego earnings to visit a dentist. Physical barriers can also be important. Dentists can establish practices wherever they like and this has led to an uneven distribution of services (Lennon, 1981). General practitioner to population ratios in England in 1986 ranged from about 1:2300 in north-west London to about 1:4200 in the West Midlands. Also the majority of practices are clustered in the more affluent areas, thus making a dental visit more difficult for those patients relying on public transport (O'Mullane and Robinson, 1977). Leichter (1980) identified three major problems in service provision:

1 There is an uneven geographical distribution of resources.
2 There are fewer health care resources in poor areas than affluent ones.
3 Many priorities are determined on political and professional grounds and are derived from the way that health care is socially organized. For example, there is more money available for acute specialties than for patients with chronic problems which require long-term care.

Emotional barriers can also present a problem. In our culture dentistry has the reputation of being painful and it seems that some people are reluctant to visit a dentist because they expect to experience pain, as discussed in Chapter 3. Another type of emotional barrier was found in Smith and Sheiham's (1980) study of elderly people. Some of those who would have liked to receive treatment had not tried to obtain it because they felt they were 'too old', while many who were in pain did not want to 'waste the dentist's time'. These feelings of low personal worth and that dental care is not 'worth it' may be important barriers for many elderly people.

Beliefs about illness and disease
Another way of looking at the discrepancy between need and demand is to consider people's norms and beliefs. Many of the issues mentioned earlier when illness behaviour was discussed are relevant here. On the one hand, an individual is unlikely to seek help if he or she does not

consider symptoms to be important. Some potentially serious dental problems do not cause severe pain, being rather insidious in nature. For example, periodontal disease can develop gradually, not giving symptoms until the teeth become loose. An unattended periapical abscess can develop into a chronic infection and ultimately a cyst which could compromise other teeth and the bony support. But if an individual is not aware of these facts and the role of screening, preventive action will not be taken. Even if pain is experienced, it may be tolerated. Many people accommodate to low-grade dental pain or a bad taste in the mouth and an impaired appearance.

One of the most widely used models for explaining preventive care is the *Health Belief Model* described by Rosenstock (1966). He tried to indicate the likelihood that someone would adopt a recommended health action by considering five factors:

1 Vulnerability: An individual who believes that he or she is susceptible to a disease may be more likely to take steps to avoid it.
2 Seriousness: The more serious a disease is seen to be, the greater the effort to avoid it.
3 Preventability: Those who believe that a disease can be prevented and who believe the methods available are effective may be more likely to act.
4 Salience: This belief has to do with the relative importance of preventive care. Those who believe that it is more important than other demands on time and effort may be more likely to take action.
5 Readiness: The belief that symptoms should be dealt with promptly rather than deferred to a later date.

There is much support for this model when these beliefs are related to *past* behaviour. Kegeles (1963), for example, found that employees of a company which provided free dental care were more likely to have made regular visits if they held at least one of these beliefs. However, *prospective* studies provide a very different picture. Weinstein et al. (1980) reported a study in which children were asked to participate in a programme of topical fluoride application. After the treatment and its effects had been explained, their health beliefs were measured. Unfortunately for the Health Belief Model, children who scored high on vulnerability, on seriousness and on the effectiveness of treatment were no more likely to take part. In fact, where the results showed a relationship, they were opposite to the predicted direction. It seems that general health beliefs such as these are poor predictors of future behaviour.

Cues to action—factors prompting a visit to the dentist
The above approaches to understanding why many people do not seek professional help have been criticized by some sociologists. The assumption behind them is that people would 'naturally' seek care if only there were no barriers to care, or if they understood the clinical meaning of their symptoms. Zola (1973) describes how he came to view the situation somewhat differently. While interviewing people in an outpatient department, he noted that many were attending with difficulties that

had bothered them for some considerable time. His question became 'Why are you coming *now*?' rather than 'Why didn't you come before?' He noted that many patients were attending not simply because there were reasons why they couldn't previously, but because their symptoms were beginning to interfere with their normal activities. He suggests that people often learn to accommodate themselves to their disabilities and only when this accommodation is upset in some way (which might be a worsening of a symptom or equally a new social demand) is action taken. In other words, demand for care arises when an impairment becomes a handicap. Zola identified five 'triggers' which can be used to predict when an individual would be likely to seek care:

1 Interference with daily life. People will often try to disregard symptoms because they are concerned that a disease will be serious, they might lose their job through illness, fail an exam or miss a holiday. If, however, an individual becomes handicapped by symptoms it becomes more difficult to ignore failing health and more likely that he or she will seek care.
2 Disruption of social life. Symptoms may not only begin to interfere with one's own routines but also relationships with friends, family or workmates. It is important that people feel an accepted part of a group and comments about bad breath or a missing front tooth may prompt a visit to a dentist.
3 Information from others about symptoms. Family or friends are often consulted about the meaning of symptoms before a visit to a dentist is made. If a symptom is believed to be significant the person is more likely to arrange an appointment.
4 Lifestyle changes. Many events in our lives, such as being married, leaving home or a bereavement, can result in changes in behaviour. This can affect visiting patterns in two ways. One is that an individual may decide to seek care because they wish to remedy a symptom that has been present for some time but could pose a threat to their enjoyment or sense of well-being at a future event. For instance someone might make an appointment for a scale and polish before a marriage. Another way in which lifestyle changes are important is that they can make accommodation to symptoms more difficult. A person might be coping with some low-grade dental pain for several weeks or months but a severe negative event (such as a bereavement) might reduce their resources to the extent that they are no longer able to cope with the pain.
5 Symptom reassessment. People can find that over time symptoms become worse. Grumbling pain from a tooth once a week may change into sharp pains every other day, thus prompting a dental visit. Reassessing symptoms can also be undertaken by setting deadlines, as in: 'if my gums are still bleeding in 3 days then I will definitely see a dentist'.

These factors amount to what Kleinman (1980) has called a lay 'explanatory model' of illness and responses to it. Such explanatory models are culturally specific and may conflict quite fundamentally with professional models of illness and health care. Such differences have several implications for dental practitioners. One implication is that they will see only a proportion of the disease in the community. Another implication is that it is often the degree of disability and handicap, rather than objective pathology, which prompts the visit. Some dentists argue that it is the handicap which requires treatment, not the disease.

The dental profession

The term 'profession' is an interesting one from a sociological point of view. It has been argued that professionals have a unique role in society because much of their work involves important values such as health, justice and education and is therefore essential for the well-being of all social groups (Parsons, 1952). Thus their work could be expected to command high material rewards and prestige. However this view is not shared by all. Some sociologists have suggested that professional groups have an inordinately high degree of control over the people they treat which can work to their own benefit rather than that of the public. A key issue is the legal right held by some professional groups to test the competence of prospective members and thereby control the number and type of practitioners in a particular field (Friedson, 1986). Johnson (1972) suggested that professionals should be viewed as a group of workers who have been particularly successful in carving out specific areas of the labour market and then excluding competition. In sociological terms, being a dental professional does not simply mean being an altruistic educated member of a society who has learned specialized duties in order to be helpful to others. It also involves a number of rights (e.g. to draw boundaries around the subject matter and determine membership) and obligations (e.g. to work to an ethical code). The following list is an amalgamation of characteristics of professions as discussed by Millerson (1964) and Dawson (1986):

1. A period of extensive training which involves the mastery of skills based on theoretical knowledge.
2. The right to monitor their own educational standards and restrict entry into the profession.
3. The freedom to regulate themselves through a licensing system and a code of ethical conduct.
4. A theme of public service and altruism.
5. Government legislation which serves to define and protect the privileges of the profession's members.

Thus a professional person is both a supplier of a service supervised for the benefit of patients and a part of a group which attempts to maintain its position against competition. There is little doubt that the 'professionalization' of dentistry has resulted in an improvement in the skill and training of practitioners, but there are many aspects of dentistry which bear closer scrutiny. This is the purpose of this section of the chapter.

Training into the dental profession

The process of becoming a dentist can be said to begin at a very early age. Just as families transmit values about the importance of dental health, so too do parents have expectations about the eventual occupations of their children. Students from lower socioeconomic groups are overwhelmingly under-represented in medical and dental schools. Most dental students come from families where the parents are financially well off, giving children access to schools where further education is highly valued. As mentioned earlier in the chapter, children in turn take on these values during the process of learning or socialization.

Socialization in dental school
The bulk of a student's undergraduate and postgraduate socialization into dentistry involves the acquisition of specialist knowledge and technical skills, but this is only part of the process. Students also learn about the ways that dentists are expected to behave and dress in front of patients. They are expected to gain an appropriate professional attitude towards their work, and so on. Some aspects of socialization are informal, as when a teacher mentions that a white coat is not as clean as it might be, or when students watch interactions between staff members and patients. Other socialization pressures are formal, as when students learn about the legislation passed by governments or professional organizations.

Research on the effects of socialization on values and norms can be performed by either following the same group of students through their course (called a longitudinal design) or by looking at different groups of students from different years (called a cross-sectional design). Steinberg (1973) used a cross-sectional design to chart the changes in students' attitudes during their course. Students were asked how they felt about a number of statements, rating them on a scale between 'not at all wrong' to 'extremely wrong'. One statement was 'refusing to treat a patient who owes you money'. One-fifth of first year students said this was not at all wrong, but 55–60% felt this in later years. Responses to 'failing to help the poor and needy' also showed changes: 43% of the first-years but 26% of the final-year students believed this to be extremely wrong. Another statement concerned profesional ethics: 'would it be right to criticize colleages when you believe them wrong?'. While 72% of first-years believed this to be not at all wrong, 37% of final-year students believed so. Eli (1984) found similar results in a longitudinal study. As students moved through the course they became more 'cynical' and concerned with the material benefits of dentistry. The value they placed on intrinsic rewards (e.g.'interest in the work' and 'opportunity to help others') declined. However after 8 years of practice following graduation the value of intrinsic rewards had risen again, while financial rewards became less important. Idealism had returned.

The dental profession—does it help?

There is no doubt that the dental profession has made a major contribution to the health and well-being of the general population. Associations of dental professionals have been the main proponents of fluoridation of the water supply and have encouraged the used of fluoride toothpaste. The preventive messages are agreed upon by the profession and, if implemented by individuals, would result in the control of periodontal disease and caries (Levine, 1989). However, some qualifications need to be placed on the assumption that everything that the profession recommends is helpful. As in other areas of health care, criticisms have been made of dentistry and the advice practitioners offer.

Treatment or prevention?
One criticism is that dentistry is primarily treatment oriented. During undergraduate teaching, students typically learn much more about how to treat already present disease than to assist in preventing it. Despite the realization that many diseases are due to how people behave, most contact between dentists and their patients involves physical interventions. The suggestion that dentists emphasize clinical interventions is supported by Eddie (1984) who noted that regular dental attenders received treatment in four out of every five review visits. She suggests that if the level of treatment could be reduced by the dental profession adopting a more preventive philosophy then the dental visit might become more of a true screening procedure and be seen as a less daunting prospect by potential patients.

This is reflected in what Croucher (1989) has called the 'performance gap'. He highlighted the discrepancy between dentists' clinical and preventive input when treating periodontal disease. Although patients were offered high quality clinical care, the dentists spent little time in helping patients to improve their oral health. Any treatment regime that does not fully explain the role of plaque in the aetiology of periodontal problems and does not offer practical advice on improving oral hygiene will fail. In the same way, restoring carious lesions without offering advice on the control of dietary sugars is not in the patient's best interests (DHSS, 1986).

The emphasis on clinical intervention rather than prevention may owe much to the way dentists are paid. The most common method of payment is the fee for item system whereby dentists are remunerated for work carried out, and the fees are negotiated between the professional and governments or insurance companies. Such a payment system rewards interventions since it encourages dentists to look for work (Dowell et al., 1983). This may in the long term be detrimental to a patient's oral health. Funding agencies have attempted to control costs by imposing constraints on high cost items such as crowns and bridges or increasing the financial contribution made by patients (Bailit et al., 1979; Bailit, 1986).

One way to resolve these problems is to move to a capitation system of payment. Under capitation the dentist is paid a fixed annual fee for maintaining the oral health of each patient. The advantages claimed are that capitation gives the dentist more clinical freedom, promotes prevention, encourages innovation and removes the financial incentive to overprescribe which is inherent in the fee for item system (Schoen, 1973). Some have argued that this new system will, in turn, result in supervised neglect, whereby dentists will tend not to intervene until a late stage in disease development. This could possibly compromise the survival of a tooth or the supporting tissues. A study by Olsen and Chetelat (1979) did note that fewer restorations and extractions were offered to patients by dentists working under a capitation scheme than those working under a fee for item system, but supervised neglect was not a problem. In the UK, the Department of Health commissioned the largest study to date on the potential value of capitation as a way of paying dentists to treat children. The study did not show that capitation was necessarily a cheaper option, but capitation dentists restored carious teeth at a later state in the disease process and offered more preventive advice (Coventry et al., 1989). The UK government has subsequently adopted a capitation scheme for use in the National Health Service for the treatment of children. Whether such a payment system is adopted elsewhere is conjecture, but it is clear that patients are becoming more aware of their oral health and are less prepared to accept clinical interventions without explanation. In industrialized countries this may be due in part to the oversupply of dentists which has increased competition. Many dentists are now offering health care rather than treatment (Wotman and Goldman, 1982).

The decision to treat

The dental profession has been criticized for the emphasis on treatment in other ways. It is important to note that the decision to intervene, and how to intervene, is rarely made on clinical criteria alone. Not only might there be financial and ethical considerations, but treatment decisions are made within a social context which will influence the decision.

Ethical issues
To a reader new to the field of ethics, it may seem that dentists have little need to be concerned with this aspect of their practice. In the popular view, ethics are mainly concerned with such major issues as abortion, euthanasia and, more recently, in vitro fertilization. However, ethics are as important in dentistry as in medicine. Perhaps the most obvious example has been the concern expressed by the media, consumer groups and government (Downer, 1988) that dentists were overprescribing restorative care. A committee was set up in 1984 by the Minister of Health in the UK to consider the problem of unnecessary dental treatment. The committee reported that there was a small but significant and unacceptable amount of deliberate unnecessary treatment in the British dental service, and a larger amount attributable to an out-of-date treatment philosophy (DHSS, 1986). Overtreatment may, in part, be due to more and more dentists chasing a pool of patients which is decreasing in size due to the general improvement in oral health.

However, dental ethics have a broader scope than overprescribing. Every consultation between a health professional and a patient has ethical implications but they are particularly important when considering treatment decisions. Training in ethics involves four main aspects of care:

1 *The aims of care:* The main aim of health care is beneficence—to act in the patient's best interests. Although it is also important to act in such as way as to do no harm, beneficence is the underlying basis of patients' trust in professionals.
2 *Value of life*: This principle concerns the value we hold for people, simply because they are human beings. Intrinsic worth does not change with age or the presence of a handicap, nor with social standing. The relative value of human over non-human life is, however, open to analysis and debate.
3 *Autonomy and consent:* This refers to everyone's right to determine their future without external constraints. Patients are in a vulnerable position and do not possess the specialist knowledge and expertise of a dentist. Nevertheless it is the patient's illness, not the dentist's, and the professional's role is to help rather than to expect obedience. Although this is clear, other related issues are not. In some instances a patient may not be capable of autonomy, being unable to give consent to treatment. Also, a patient's autonomy could affect the freedom and rights of others.
4 *Truth and integrity:* The fourth principle concerns the importance of truth-telling. On the one hand, there are the ethical obligations not to mislead patients, to keep faith with any stated intentions and to ensure confidentiality. A dentist would, for example, be under an ethical obligation to disclose any financial advantages to him or herself when a course of treatment is recommended. But again there can be exceptions, such as when a dentist has a duty to society or other patients which overrides confidentiality.

Ethical considerations involve the processes of examining and weighing up the importance of these principles in particular situations (Johnson, 1990). There is often no one right answer when an ethical dilemma is faced because in a given situation one principle (such as autonomy) might conflict with another (such as beneficence). The skill lies in making a considered analysis of the ethical implications of actions.

Social influences
Thus, treatment decisions are influenced by financial and ethical considerations. They are also influenced by current social values. On the one hand, there are prevailing professional views about treatment which fall within the professional 'explanatory model'. However these are not always supported by research evidence. The theory of focal infections, which was widely believed between 1918 and 1940, held that even mildly diseased teeth could be responsible for a large number of systemic disorders. This resulted in the widespread extraction of teeth (Burt, 1978). More recently, Sheiham (1977) has drawn the profession's attention to the fact that the guidelines on screening have little scientific validity and that the recommended goal of 6-monthly inspections may deter some individuals from seeking routine care.

There can also be sizeable discrepancies between lay and professional views about the need for treatment. The treatment of malocclusion provides a good example. Common sense might predict that a good indicator of the decision to seek orthodontic treatment would be a dental index of occlusion. However this seems to hold only for severe malocclusions and then only when irregularities are clearly visible. While many people with malocclusions are not satisfied with the state of their dentition, this must be set against the sizeable proportion of people with objectively minor irregularities who are also dissatisfied (Lewit and Virolainen, 1968; Ingervall and Hedegard, 1974). Many people whom dentists believe require care do not seek it. In one study of 18-year-olds, about 25% were considered to need urgent or moderately urgent care, yet only 3% wanted it (Ingervall et al., 1978).

This discrepancy between those conditions that dentists consider require treatment and patients' views suggests that the two groups are using different criteria or have different values. This suggestion was supported in one study (Prahl-Andersen et al., 1979) in which lay-people, dentists and orthodontists were shown drawings and photographs of children with various dentofacial morphologies. Almost without exception the professionals were more likely to say that the dentitions were abnormal and needed treatment. There is also considerable variation in professionals' judgements. Jago (1974) reviewed several epidemiological studies of dental malocclusion, finding that rates ranged from 1.4 to 83.6% depending, it seemed, on the criteria used by the investigators as well as on the populations studied. Jago argues that malocclusion is primarily a value judgement and there is no ideal or objective standard which can be used to determine need for treatment. While functional difficulty is often cited as a reason for orthodontic care, there is little evidence that it makes any difference to the severity of periodontal disease (Ramfijord, 1987). As discussed in Chapter 6, there is also little evidence that it improves patients' self-esteem.

These findings indicate that social and psychological factors as well as clinical ones are important in treatment decisions. One influence comes from within the profession itself. When Shaw et al. (1979) asked mothers why they were seeking orthodontic care for their children, 70% said it was a dentist who first suggested that the children needed treatment. Another influence is cultural views of attractiveness. One of the better predictors of demand for orthodontic care is patients' (or their parents') belief that the malocclusion detracts from physical attractiveness (Crawford, 1974; Albino et al., 1981). Some parents consider malocclusion to be a social and psychological handicap. Shaw et al. (1979) found that some three-quarters of parents of orthodontic patients believed that straightening the teeth would make their child more attractive and that orthodontic treatment was important or very important for success in a future occupation. This seems to be related to socioeconomic status: Kenealy et al. (1989) found that children from middle-class backgrounds were over three times more likely to enter treatment for minor malocclusions than children from working class backgrounds.

Social influences are relevant for non-cosmetic treatment decisions as well. The decision to state positively that a patient requires a replacement filling, has a carious cavity, requires periodontal surgery or has a TMJD worthy of further investigation depends to a large extent on the individual dentist. His or her decision to treat will depend on such factors as clinical experience, contact with other dentists and attendance at postgraduate courses. It is clear however that there is a wide variation between dentists as to what constitutes disease (Kay et al., 1988) or a failed restoration (Elderton and Nuttal, 1983). Kay and Blinkhorn (1987) examined the processes involved in the decision to extract teeth. Although the extent of dental disease was clearly important, the decision was not necessarily directly related to disease. For instance, they found that dentists were more likely to take radiographs in order to complement their diagnosis that an extraction was needed if the patient was a regular attender than an irregular one. This seemed to be related to the dentists' higher motivation to give a more thorough type of clinical care to regular attenders, since a radiograph provides additional information which may indicate that the tooth can be saved.

Iatrogenic illness
A further professional issue concerns the problem of iatrogenic illness (*iatros*, Greek for physician; *genesis*, meaning origin). Some writers have argued that there are many aspects of medical and dental care which work to the detriment of patients. Illich (1977), a leading proponent of this view, argues that the health professions can have negative effects in several ways. Clinical iatrogenic illness refers to the ways in which treatments can be 'sickening agents'. Some examples of these have been mentioned previously. The widespread extraction of teeth due to the unproven theory of focal infection left a great many people edentulous. The 1986 DHSS report which indicated that there was a small but unacceptable degree of unnecessary treatment under the National Health Service is another example. Nuttal (1984) reported that regular attenders had twice as many tooth surfaces filled as infrequent attenders and that much of this clinical work involved replacing restorations for no obvious reason. Elderton and Nuttal (1983) suggest that many practitioners need to review their replacement criteria critically and spend more time on trying to help patients prevent dental disease.

Illich also argues that health professionals increase the incidence of disease by portraying themselves as having curative abilities. The proportion of the national wealth devoted to health care has been increasing more quickly than any other sector of the economy. Since most dental diseases can be prevented at a much lower cost, perhaps a greater proportion of resources should be aimed at encouraging people to control their sugar intake, brush effectively and ensure an adequate intake of fluoride. The emphasis on restorative dentistry may lead people to believe that their oral health problems can be solved when the time comes, making them less likely to take preventive measures in the short-term. When the dental profession takes responsibility for health, it is argued, individuals are not encouraged to look after themselves.

Such criticisms have worried some dentists (e.g. Carrington, 1986) who feel that their professional value is being undermined. Elderton (1986) has stressed that this is not the case, but that critical evaluation of the restorative philosophy of dental care has shown that in many instances dentistry as it is currently practised may not be in patients' best interests.

The profession's future

The studies outlined in this chapter are of more than academic interest to the reader. The changing patterns of disease found by epidemiological studies will require substantial changes in the way dental professionals work in the years to come. In the past, the major oral problem of caries has meant that the main focus of dental education has been on the learning of techniques to restore and extract teeth. The World Health Organization (1990) argues that the steep decline in caries and edentulousness will require a change in emphasis towards other oral problems if the profession is to thrive. In some cases this will involve a greater concern with high-technology interventions, such as the use of osseointegrated implants and regenerative techniques, while in other cases it will be a greater emphasis on social and psychological aspects of practice. The relationship between the dentist and the patient will be thrown into sharper focus and it is becoming increasingly important to find ways of encouraging infrequent attenders to visit more regularly. In part, this can be accomplished through the alleviation of anxiety and expectations of pain. Consideration of such aspects of dental care is the aim of the following chapters.

Summary

One of the principal aims of sociologists and psychologists is to provide explanations of social behaviour. In sociology the notions of values (collective beliefs), norms (ideas about how people should behave) and socialization (the process of learning values and norms) are central. Dentists and lay-people can hold different values and norms about oral health. These differences apply not only to the importance of preventive care but also to such basic questions as the need for treatment and definitions of ill health. It seems that dentists place most value on the absence and treatment of disease but for many lay-people questions about disability and handicap are more significant.

Epidemiological studies of disease have found that the prevalence of dental ill health is related to socioeconomic level, which in turn is related to differences in behaviour and provision of services. The substantial decline in caries found in western societies recently may be largely due to fluoridation of the water supply and toothpaste. This has important implications for future dental practice.

Currently, professional training is mainly concerned with teaching the techniques and skills needed for restorative care, but there is a wide variation between dentists in treatment practices. Financial, ethical and social influences as well as clinical criteria affect treatment decisions. Training in dentistry involves learning the values of the profession, as well as the skills. Some of these values have been called into question by dentists who have are concerned their appropriateness.

Practice implications

1 People can have very different views from dentists about dental health and ill health. Such differences need to be kept in mind when explaining the professional view.

2 Socioeconomic level has many important effects and may affect treatment decisions. The costs of attendance, such as having to take time off work, and the relative importance of dental health will need to be taken into account.
3 Consider the amount of time and effort put into preventive care as opposed to restorative work.

Suggested reading

David Locker's book *Behavioural Sciences and Dentistry* (London, Tavistock, 1989) covers the sociological aspects of dental care in more detail, while Helman C. *Culture, Health and Illness* (Bristol, Wright, 1984) discusses cross-cultural views of illness.

References

Abercrombie N., Warde A. (1988) *Contemporary British Society*. Oxford: Blackwell.
Albino J.E., Cunat J., Fox R., Lewis E., Slakter M., Tedesco L. (1981) Variables discriminating individuals who seek orthodontic treatment. *J. Dent. Res.* **60,**1661–7.
Attwood D., Salapata J., Blinkhorn A. (1990) Comparison of the dental health of 12 year old children living in Athens and Glasgow. *Int. Dent. J.* **40,**117–21.
Bailit H. (1986) Future financing of health care. *J. Dent. Educ.* **50,**119–24.
Bailit H., Raskin M., Reisine S., Chiriboga D. (1979) Controlling the cost of dental care.*Am. J. Public Health Dent.* **69,**699–703.
Beal J.F. (1990) The dental health of black and ethnic minority communities. *Community Dent. Health* **7,**121–2.
Bergner M., Bobbitt B. (1981) The Sickness Impact Profile: development and final revision of a health status measure. *Med. Care* **19,**787–805.
Blinkhorn A.S. (1989) Promoting dietary changes in order to control dental caries. *J. Inst. Dent. Educ.* **27,**179–86.
Blinkhorn A.S., Hastings G., Leathar D. (1983) Attitudes towards dental care among young people in Scotland. *Br. Dent. J.* **155,**311–3.
Blomberg S., Linquist L. (1983) Psychological reactions to edentulousness and treatment with jawbone-anchored bridges. *Acta Psychiatr. Scand.* **68,**251–62.
Burt B. (1978) Influences for change in the dental health status of populations; an historical perspective. *J. Public Health Dent.* **38,**272–88.
Burt B. (1985) The future of caries decline. *J. Public Health Dent.* **45,**261–9.
Carlsson G.E. (1976) Symptoms of mandibular dysfunction in complete denture wearers. *J. Dent.* **4,**265–70.
Carrington H.B. (1986) Reflections on Elderton's 'Restoration 85'. *Br. Dent. J.* **160,**36–7.
Coventry P., Holloway P., Lennon M., Mellor A., Worthington H. (1989) A trial of a capitation system of payment for the treatment of children in the general dental service. *Community Dent. Health* **6,** suppl. 1.
Craft M., Croucher R. (1980) *The 16 to 20 Study* London: Health Education Council.
Crawford T.P. (1974) A multiple regression analysis of patient cooperation during treatment. *Am. J. Orthod.* **65,**436–7.
Croucher R. (1989) *The Performance Gap*. London: Health Education Authority.
Cushing A., Sheiham A., Maizels J. (1986) Developing socio-dental indicators – the social impact of dental disease. *Community Dent. Health* **3,**3–17.
Dawson S. (1986) *Analysing Organizations*.London: Macmillan.
DHSS (1986) *Report of a Committee of Inquiry into Unnecessary Dental Treatment*. London: HMSO.

Douglass C.W., Cole K. (1979) The supply of dental manpower in the United States. *Am. J. Dent. Educ.* **43**,287–302.

Dowell T.B., Holloway P., Keshani D., Clerehugh V. (1983) Do dentists fill teeth unnecessarily? *Br. Dent. J.* **155**,247–9.

Downer M.C. (1988) Expectations for oral health in Great Britain and the response of the dental care system. *J. Public Health Dent.* **48**,98–102.

Eddie S. (1984) Frequency of attendance in the general dental service in Scotland. *Br. Dent. J.* **157**,267–70.

Elderton R.J. (1986) For debate. *Br. Dent. J.* **160**,37–8.

Elderton R.J., Nuttal N. (1983) Variation amongst dentists in planning treatment. *Br. Dent. J.* **154**,201–6.

Eli I. (1984) Professional socialization into dentistry: a longitudinal analysis of changes in students' expected professional rewards. *Soc. Sci. Med.*, pp. 297–302.

Elkin F., Handel G. (1972) *The Child and Society. The Process of Socialization.* 2nd ed.n New York, Random House.

Friedson E. (1986) The medical profession in transition. In *Applications of Social Science to Clinical Medicine and Health Policy* (Aiken L., Mechanic D., eds) New Brunswick, Rutgers University Press.

General Dental Council (1990) *Guidance on the Teaching of Behavioural Sciences.* London: GDC.

Gift H.C. (1985) Utilization of professional dental services. In *Social Sciences and Dentistry* (Cohen K.L., Bryant P., eds) London: Quintessence.

Gray P.G., Todd J., Slack G., Bulman J. (1970) *Adult Dental Health in England and Wales in 1968.* London: HMSO.

Hannay D. (1988) *Lecture Notes on Medical Sociology.* London: Blackwell.

Haraldson T., Karlsson U., Carlsson G. (1979) Bite force and oral function in complete denture wearers. *J. Oral Rehabil.* **6**,41–8.

Heyink J.W., Heezen J., Schaub R. (1986) Dentist and patient appraisal of complete dentures in a Dutch elderly population. *Community Dent. Oral Epidemiol.* **14**, 323–6.

Hochstein J.R., Athanasopoulos D., Larkins J. (1968) Poverty area under the microscope. *Am. J. Public Health* **58**,1815–27.

Illich I. (1977) *Limits to Medicine.* Harmondsworth, Pelican.

Ingervall B., Hedegard B. (1974) Awareness of malocclusion and desire for orthodontic treatment in 18 year old Swedish men. *Acta Orthodont. Scand.* **32**, 93–101.

Ingervall B., Mohlin B., Thilander B. (1978) Prevalence and awareness of malocclusion in Swedish men. *Community Dent. Oral Epidemiol.* **6**,308–14.

Jago J.D. (1974) The epidemiology of dental occlusion: a critical appraisal. *J. Public Health Dent.* **34**, 80–93.

Jarman B. (1984) Identification of underprivileged areas. *Br. Med. J.* **286**,1705–9.

Johnson A.(1990) *Pathways in Medical Ethics.* London: Edward Arnold.

Johnson T. (1972) *Professions and Power.* London: Macmillan.

Kay E.J., Blinkhorn A. (1987) Some factors related to dentists' decisions to extract teeth. *Community Dent. Health* **4**,3–9.

Kay E.J., Watts A., Paterson R., Blinkhorn A. (1988) Preliminary investigation into the validity of dentists' decisions to restore occlusal surfaces of permanent teeth. *Community Dent. Oral Epidemiol.* **16**,91–4.

Kegeles S.S. (1963) Some motives for seeking preventive health care. *J. Am. Dent. Assoc.* **67**,90–8.

Kenealy P., Frude N., Shaw W. (1989) The effects of social class on the uptake of orthodontic treatment. *Br. J. Orthodont.* **16**,107–11.

Kent G. (1983) Psychology in the dental curriculum. *Br. Dent. J.* **154**,106–9.

Kleinman A. (1980) *Patients and Healers in the Context of Culture.* Berkeley, University of California Press.

Laher M.H.E. (1990) A comparison between dental caries, gingival health and dental service usage in Bangladeshi and white Caucasian children aged 7, 9, 11, 13 and 15 years residing in an inner city area of London: U.K. *Community Dent. Health* **7**,157–63.

Leichter H. (1980) *A Comparative Approach to Policy Analysis. Health Care Policy in Four Nations.* Cambridge: Cambridge University Press.
Lennon M.A. (1981) The organization of dental services in the United Kingdom. In *Dental Public Health* (2nd edn) (Slack G.L., ed) Bristol: Wright.
Levine R. (ed.) (1989) *The Scientific Basis of Dental Health Education.* 3rd edn. London: Health Education Authority.
Lewit D.W., Virolainen K. (1968) Conformity and independence in adolescents' motivation for orthodontic treatment. *Child Dev.* **39,**1189–200.
Locker D. (1988) Measuring oral health: a conceptual framework. *Community Dent. Health* **5,**3–18.
Locker D., Slade G. (1988) Prevalence of symptoms associated with temporomandibular disorders in a Canadian population. *Community Dent. Oral Epidemiol.* **16,**310–3.
Magnusson T. (1980) Prevalence of recurrent headache and mandibular dysfunction in patients with unsatisfactory dentures *Community Dent. Oral Epidemiol.* **8,**159–64.
McKeown T. (1979) *The Role of Medicine.* Oxford: Blackwell.
Metz A.S., Richards L. (1967) Children's preventive dental visits. *J. Am. Coll. Dent.* **34,**204–12.
Millerson G. (1964) *The Qualifying Associations.* London: Routledge.
Moosbrucker J., Jong A. (1969) Racial similarities and differences in family dental care patterns. *Public Health Rep.* **84,**721–7.
Nuttal N. (1984) General dental service treatment received by frequent and infrequent dental attenders in Scotland. *Br. Dent. J.* **156,**363–6.
Olsen E.D., Chetalat G. (1979) Dental capitation programs. A comparison of delivery systems. *J. Calif. Dent. Assoc.* **7,**47–50.
O'Mullane D.M., Robinson M. (1977) The distribution of dentists and the uptake of dental treatment by school children in England. *Community Dent. Oral Epidemiol.* **5,**156–9.
OPCS (1980) *Classification of Occupations.* London: HMSO.
OPCS (1986) The 1983 update on adult dental health from OPCS. *Br. Dent. J.* **160,**246–53.
OPCS (1990) *Standard Occupational Classification.* London: HMSO.
Opler M.K., Singer S. (1956) Ethnic differences in behaviour and psycho-pathology. *Int. J. Psychiatry* **2,**11–22.
Parsons T. (1952) *The Social System.* London: Tavistock and Free Press.
Peter J., Chinsky R. (1974) Sociological aspects of cleft palate adults. l: Marriage. *Cleft Palate J.* **11,**259–309.
Prahl-Andersen B., Boersma H., van der Linden F., Moore A. (1979) Perceptions of dentofacial morphology by laypersons, general dentists and orthodontists. *J. Am. Dent. Assoc.* **98,** 209–12.
Ramfijord S.O. (1987) Periodontal significance of orthodontic therapy. In *The 1987 Dental Annual* (Derrick D.D., ed.). Wright: Bristol.
Reisine S.T. (1988) The effects of pain and oral health on the quality of life. *Community Dent. Health* **5,**63–8.
Rosenstock I.M. (1966) Why people use health services. *Millbank Mem. Fund Q.* **4,**92–124.
Schoen M.A. (1973) Observation of selected dental services under two prepayment mechanisms. *Am. J. Public Health* **63,**727–31.
Shaw W.C., Gabe M., Jones B. (1979) The expectations of orthodontic patients in South Wales and St. Louis, Missouri. *Br. J. Orthodont.* **6,**203–5.
Sheiham A. (1977) Is there a scientific basis for six monthly dental examinations? *Lancet* **201,**442–4.
Smith J.P. (1977) Observer variation in the clinical diagnosis of mandibular pain dysfunction syndrome. *Community Dent. Oral. Epidemiol* **5,**91–3.
Smith J.M., Sheiham A. (1979) How dental conditions handicap the elderly. *Community Dent. Oral Epidemiol* **7,**305–10.
Smith J.M., Sheiham A. (1980) Dental treatment needs and demands of an elderly population in England. *Community Dent. Oral Epidemiol.* **8,**360–4.
Steinberg D.N. (1973) Changes in attitudes of dental students *J. Dent. Educ.* **37,**36–41.

Todd J.E., Walker A.M. (1980) *Adult Dental Health (Vol 1). England and Wales, 1968–1978.* London: HMSO.

Townsend P., Davidson N. (1982) *The Black Report.* Middlesex: Penguin.

Weinstein M., Kegeles S., Lund A. (1980) Children's health beliefs and acceptance of a dental prevention activity. *J. Health Soc. Behav.* **21,**59–74.

Williams S.A. (1984) Infant feeding practices and dental health. *Community Dent. Health* **1,**78 (Abstract).

Williams S.A., Fairpo C. (1988) Cultural variations in oral hygiene practices among infants resident in an inner city area. *Community Dent. Health.* **5,**265–71.

Woolgrove J., Cumberbach G., Gelbier S. (1987) Understanding dental attendance behaviour. *Community Dent. Health* **4,**215–21.

World Health Organization (1980) *International Classification of Impairments, Disabilities and Handicaps.* Geneva: WHO.

World Health Organization (1990) *Educational Imperatives for Oral Health Personnel: Change or Decay?* Geneva: WHO.

Wotman S., Goldman H. (1982) Pressures on the dental care system in the United States. *Am. J. Public Health* **72,**684–9.

Zola I. (1973) Pathways to the doctor: from person to patient. *Soc. Sci. Med.* **7,**677–89.

Chapter 2

Prevention: The educational and behavioural viewpoints

In the previous chapter some of the important sociological aspects of dentistry were discussed. The central theme was that dental care is always provided within a social and cultural context which affects both the definition of dental disease and the likelihood that an individual will consult a dentist. Lay and professional people may have very different beliefs about what problems merit professional care. In this chapter we turn to more specific aspects of the complex area of the prevention of oral disease. In particular, the interest here is in ways that people can be encouraged to engage in preventive care, both at home and by regular visits to the dentist. One reason for the concern about prevention is the increasing recognition that much of the disease seen by a practitioner is due to aspects of lifestyle, especially diet, the use of a fluoride toothpaste and the efficient removal of dental plaque.

There are two main strands to the research discussed here. One emphasizes educational objectives. The argument is that once people become aware of the importance of preventive care, and how to achieve it, they will be much more likely to change their diet, brush effectively and seek regular oral health screening. Thus interventions which increase knowledge and skills should have a noticeable impact on health. The other strand emphasizes motivation. Many psychologists argue that although knowledge and skills are important and necessary conditions for preventive care, they may not be in themselves sufficient. Unless people experience some positive consequences for engaging in preventive behaviour they are unlikely to go to the expense and effort involved. To anticipate the conclusions of this chapter, it seems that both educational and motivational approaches must be taken if preventive programmes are to work. The final section of the chapter provides suggestions for designing a preventive programme which can be adapted for the use of individual patients.

The educational approach

Put at its simplest, the educational approach holds that people do not engage in preventive care because they are either not aware of the importance of doing so or do not have the necessary ability and skills.

Several surveys have shown that there is a surprising lack of knowledge about hygiene practices in the general population. In one sample of dental patients, 63% reported that they had never heard of the word 'plaque', 29% could not remember having been instructed on how to brush their teeth, and none could remember having been told of the significance of the stickiness or frequency of eating sweets (Linn, 1974). In a study of mothers of preschool children, only 20% reported having received any advice on how to care for their children's teeth (Blinkhorn, 1978). Another survey of 16–20-year-olds indicated that 25% thought that it was 'natural' for their gums to bleed during brushing (Craft and Croucher, 1980). While it is important to realize that these results are based on respondents' memories (perhaps they had been told but had forgotten), these studies suggest that there is a significant lack of accurate information about dental care. It may be that this is partly responsible for the problem.

Experiments on educational programmes

There have been numerous attempts to confirm the hypothesis that behaviour will change after exposure to an educational programme. The usual method has been first to select a sample of patients, randomly divide them into two groups, and then provide the education (perhaps through films or discussion) to one group but not to the other. The purpose of this random assignment is to ensure that any relevant variables, such as income level, social class or educational attainment, will be equally represented in the two groups.

In a good study the patients who are not exposed to the educational package (the control group) would be treated in as similar a way as possible as those given extra knowledge and skills (the experimental group). The control group would also be shown films or engaged in discussion, but these would concentrate on aspects unrelated to the specifics of dental education. By making the treatment of the two groups the same except for the variable under study, other possible interpretations of the results are ruled out. The control group would then serve as a comparison when changes in behaviour or oral health are monitored after the intervention. In a more complex study, there could be more than two groups: perhaps two different educational programmes with different emphases could be compared to each other as well as to no intervention.

Long-term effects of educational programmes
A good example of an experiment on dental education is given by Horowitz et al. (1976). One group of children was given 10 30-minute sessions on plaque removal, being taught in small groups by a dental hygienist. They were told about plaque, how to identify it with disclosing agents, and how to remove it. Each day for the next 6 months plaque removal was practised under supervision. Disclosing agents were used regularly and the children were asked to re-brush and re-floss any remaining plaque. All of this added up to a considerable amount of time, effort and education. The comparison group of children were not given any of this extra information or practice.

Three measures of oral hygiene were taken—a plaque score, a gingival inflammation (GI) score and a caries score. These measures were taken before the programme began (called a baseline), again at the end of the treatment sessions (at 8 months) and then again 4 months later. At baseline, the two groups were similar on all measures, indicating that they were comparable to begin with. At the 8-month assessment there was a significant decline in GI scores in the education group compared to the control group. This was initially encouraging, but at 12 months there was again no difference. There was no long-term effect. Nor were there ever any differences in caries levels or the amount of plaque in the two groups.

Unfortunately, this is a typical result. The general finding of such studies has been short-term gain during the intervention but little improvement when further assessments are made several months later. It seems that people often revert to their previous behaviour when the intervention ceases. While educational programmes do influence the amount of knowledge and skill people possess, they have only a small effect on long-term behaviour.

Reasons for the failure of educational programmes
There are several possible reasons for the lack of long-term effects after educational interventions. One is that the programmes are usually work- or school-centred: encouragement and practice may be given at school, but few attempts are made to integrate these into the home environment. This may be crucial. Perhaps, too, the people in such studies become dependent on the teaching staff to remind them to brush and floss. When the programme ends so too do the constant reminders.

Another possibility is that while the educational approach provides part of the answer to changing behaviour, it is not in itself sufficient. That is, although people require information and skills, they may not have the motivation to act on this information.

This idea that education is not sufficient is supported by such studies as that of Todd et al. (1982). Although 91% of a nationwide sample agreed that regular visits to the dentist are important for keeping their teeth healthy, 43% claimed that they went to the dentist only when they were experiencing some symptoms. This discrepancy between what people know they should do and their actual behaviour may be due to motivational factors, especially the perceived consequences of their actions. This aspect of preventive care is discussed later in the chapter.

Education in practice

The practising dentist faces some common problems with educationalists in that both are concerned with increasing knowledge and skills. But here there is a greater opportunity to tailor training to the individual patient's needs. This requires thoughtful communication. General aspects of communicating with patients are taken up in detail in Chapter 7, but there are some specific aspects which are particularly related to preventive care education.

For a variety of reasons—such as the patient's level of educational attainment—it is important to make some decisions about how to present information. Misunderstandings are remarkably common between professionals and lay-people, and often information is forgotten within minutes of the end of an interview. Because of this, there have been strong recommendations to provide patients with written information—something that they can take away to read over and remind themselves of the important points of a consultation.

Written information can be useful in a variety of settings. It has been used when preparing patients for surgery and explaining the nature of various diseases as well as for getting the preventive message across. Many dentists display pamphlets in their waiting rooms, but there is a large body of evidence that such pamphlets are not understood by a substantial number of patients (Blinkhorn and Verity, 1979). Their usefulness also depends on whether they are noticed, read, believed and remembered (Ley, 1988).

Understanding text
Several factors need to be taken into account when designing material. Kanouse and Hayes-Roth (1980) list ways to increase the ease with which text can be understood. These include:

1 Using active rather than passive verbs.
2 Using concrete rather than abstract words.
3 Stating ideas explicitly rather than implicitly.
4 Using the same words consistently when referring to a disease or treatment.
5 Using numbering when presenting facts.
6 Putting old information at the beginning of a sentence, new information at the end.

The typeface is also important, as Poulton et al. (1970) point out. They provide several guidelines:

1 Type should be at least 10 point.
2 Indenting the first line of a paragraph increases speed of reading.
3 Printing in capital letters reduces speed of comprehension.
4 Printing in italics reduces speed of reading.
5 Headings will stand out better if a different typeface is used than for the text.
6 Unjustified lines are easier to read.

Reading ease
Another aspect of ease of comprehension is readability. Text with a large proportion of polysyllabic words and long sentences is difficult to read. Short sentences are much easier. One way of calculating reading ease is the Flesch formula (Flesch, 1951):

Reading ease = $206.835 - 0.846wl - 1.05sl$

where *wl* = number of syllables per 100 words (word length) and *sl* = number of words per sentence (sentence length).

A score below 60 is considered fairly difficult, below 50 difficult. For material designed for children, the score should be much higher, perhaps 90 plus.

As well as testing text for reading ease, it would also be important to select terms which could be understood by most readers. For example, the word 'plaque' is short but few people understand its meaning. If such terms are to be used they need explanation.

Expertise
Not only must care be taken in deciding what is given to patients, but also in selecting who gives the information. Patients are more likely to accept and follow advice when it is given by someone whom they consider to be an expert, rather than by someone who is less qualified. This principle was tested by asking dentists, dental assistants and receptionists to give patients the same brief speech: 'There is a new dental care booklet I think you should read. It is free of charge if you just fill out this card with your name and address and drop it in a mail box'. Each card was covertly marked to indicate which of the three individuals gave the card to the patient. In one practice, 60% of the dentist's patients returned the card, 43% of the assistant's, and 23% of the receptionist's; in the other practice the rates were 47, 27 and 13% (Levine et al., 1978). These results suggest that if a dental assistant or receptionist is to give advice then the message may need to be reinforced in some way by the dentist.

The behavioural approach

As mentioned earlier, some psychologists believe that educational approaches to preventive care have been unsuccessful because they do not take patients' motivations into account. These psychologists argue that people will take preventive actions only when they can see some kind of clear benefit for doing so, and the benefit needs to be apparent in the short term rather than some years in the future.

Behavioural analysis

The basic theory behind this approach is fairly straightforward. Antecedents of behaviour are those cues (or *stimuli*, as they are technically called) in the environment which lead us to behave in certain ways. So, for example, a person who smokes may light up directly after a meal or with every cup of coffee. Brushing is often linked with washing, so that the habitual action after washing one's face is to brush one's teeth. The likelihood that an antecedent will, in fact, come to evoke behaviour depends on the consequences of that behaviour. When someone performs an action and the consequences are rewarding, the person is likely to repeat that action. If the consequences are unfavourable, the behaviour is less likely to be repeated. A student may study a subject either because it is intrinsically rewarding or because it is necessary to pass an examination in order to qualify, and qualification is rewarding. Here, the future consequences can be said to determine the present behaviour.

Reinforcement
Psychologists use the term *reinforcer* to mean any consequence which increases the likelihood of behaviour being shown. The reinforcer could be based on primary biological needs (e.g. food, water) or on things which are not intrinsically rewarding but have become so because of past experience, called secondary reinforcers. Another distinction is between positive and negative reinforcers. A positive reinforcer is a consequence which is pleasant and increases the likelihood of behaviour when it is offered. Examples are food, money and praise. A dentist may work harder and see more patients if there is the promise of financial reward. An unpleasant event which can be avoided through some kind of action is called a negative reinforcer. The threats of failing an examination or being asked to leave a course of study are negative reinforcers. Faced with such consequences, a student may begin reading textbooks and studying in order to avoid them.

Punishment is quite a different concept from negative reinforcement. It is an unpleasant consequence which *reduces* the likelihood of behaviour being repeated. A parent who revokes a child's privileges for being naughty or a dentist who chastises a patient for eating too much sugar are both attempting, through punishment, to reduce the likelihood of these behaviours.

A way of remembering the inter-relationship between these basic principles is:

A the antecedents of behaviour;
B the behaviour itself;
C the consequences of behaviour.

Applications of a behavioural analysis

These principles have been widely applied in psychology. As an example of how they might be used in practice, consider how a dentist might react to children in the surgery. A child who is well behaved and co-operative during treatment might be praised and given a small present such as a sticky badge. For this child, there is a positive consequence for attending and co-operating. Conversely, a co-operative child may simply be examined, treated if necessary, and then sent home again with no reinforcement for being co-operative. For this child there are few positive consequences for helpful behaviour, so it may be less likely to occur again on the next visit. In the absence of reinforcers the co-operative behaviour could eventually become less likely or *extinguish*.

Preventive care
There are a large number of studies reporting the successful use of these principles of antecedent and consequence in a wide variety of situations. They are particularly relevant to preventive care. Zifferblat (1975) argues

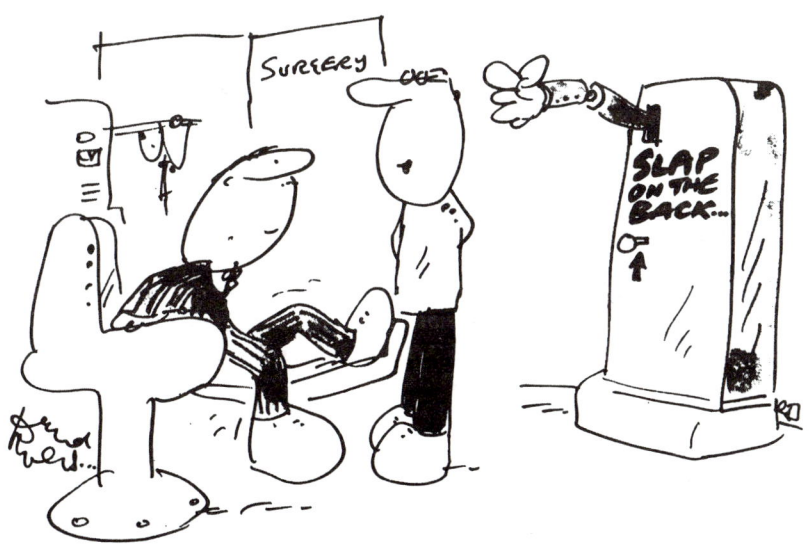

"You've been a splendid patient — stand by the machine and press the button..."
(Reproduced by permission of David Myers.)

that whether or not a patient follows advice is a function of the environmental events which immediately precede and follow the prescribed behaviour. A headache or an upset stomach, for example, would provide cues for taking medication. Similarly, if the patient can feel or observe that 'this is the time to take my medication' or 'this is the time to brush and floss my teeth' easily and unambiguously, compliance would tend to be high. If however there is no obvious signal or antecedent the probability of compliance would be low. This could occur if a drug or advice is given as a preventive measure: by the time the patient realizes the advice was important, it is already too late. Similarly, if the patient believes that preventive advice has positive consequences, then he or she will be likely to follow that advice. But if there are no clear and positive consequences, the behaviour could extinguish. A problem that people have when on a diet, for example, is that the positive consequences (weight loss) will be experienced sometime in the future, while the negative consequences (hunger) are experienced in the present.

There are similar difficulties for dental patients. While brushing with a fluoridated toothpaste, reducing sugar consumption and regular flossing may reduce the likelihood of caries and periodontal disease in the long run, noticeable symptoms may not appear for months or years. The most important factor in caries development is diet, particularly the amount and frequency of sugar consumption. Eating sugar has positive short-term consequences while the negative consequences are apparent only in the longer term.

From the behavioural analyst's point of view this is inherently problematic. Patients are being asked to act in order to avoid disease, but this involves a sacrifice of an immediate reward for dental health sometime in the distant future. If good preventive care is practised, the negative consequence of neglect will not be experienced. Children are most at risk because they are less likely to be concerned with long-term objectives and less able to imagine the negative consequences of poor oral health habits.

Thus the A-B-C principle is extremely relevant to preventive care in dentistry. Because brushing and dietary changes may not be inherently reinforcing, preventive care is unlikely if there is no external reason for compliance. There are two ways in which this difficulty might be overcome. One method is to provide positive reinforcements which are contingent on self-care. This approach has formed the bulk of research in this area. The second method involves making the negative consequences of poor oral health care more salient. While this has always been one aim of educational programmes, there are additional strategies which can be used which are consistent with the behavioural approach.

Providing positive reinforcements

This common-sense approach is used both by parents when praising their children for brushing or by dentists when congratulating their patients for having little plaque on their teeth. However, a psychologist would require some experimental validation of this principle some evidence that the procedure of providing external positive reinforcements for practising regular preventive measures is indeed useful. Its usefulness should be compared with other methods. If another way of changing behaviour were more effective, then this might be preferable. This part of the chapter considers these issues.

Material incentives

In experiments with children and adults, rewards are often given in the form of material goods such as toys or money rather than verbal praise. For example, Reiss et al. (1976) attempted to encourage mothers to bring their children for a dental screening. These parents were from low-income families, so that cash seemed to be an appropriate incentive. One-third of the mothers received a note giving an explanation of the screening and a request to attend with their children. Another third received this note plus two personal calls, one on the telephone and one in person. The third group received the note plus a promise of $5 if they attended. The results indicated that the cash incentive was the most effective of the three methods and was much more cost effective than the two personal calls. In another study with children themselves, those who were given small rewards for having clean teeth improved their hygiene more over the course of the study than a control group of children who were not rewarded (Martens et al., 1973).

Although these and other studies have indicated that this approach is effective, one concern about using material rewards for dental care is the possibility that once the incentives are withdrawn, the behaviour will return to previous levels or, worse, that it might cease altogether. Fortunately, there is evidence that this does not necessarily occur. In the case of the screening attendance study described above, more children in the reward group completed any necessary restorative work than in the other two groups, even though continued attendance was not rewarded financially. Similarly, in the study with children themselves, the difference between the control and incentive groups was maintained 6 months after the termination of the reward regime.

Providing material rewards can be rather expensive so it would be useful to compare it with other methods for improving preventive behaviour. In the first section of this chapter, for example, evidence that education can sometimes increase preventive care was discussed. Does reinforcement add to the effectiveness of education? This question was studied by dividing a practice's patients into two groups. One group was given an education programme about the detrimental effects of plaque, the importance of controlling it and the means of control. The patients' teeth were examined and cleaned and disclosing tablets issued so that the patients could monitor their plaque. On two later visits, further instruction and guided practice with brushing technique were given. A second group of patients was given this education programme plus an incentive: their treatment could cost up to 25% less if they were able to keep their plaque scores down.

At the end of the treatment programme, both groups of patients had lower plaque scores than at the beginning, indicating that both education alone and education plus incentive had an effect. However, the education plus incentive group showed a greater improvement: only 1 of 14 patients in the education only group reduced their plaque by 10% or more while 15 of the 17 patients in the education plus incentive group did so. Furthermore, 6 months later the improvement for the incentive plus education group was maintained over the initial baseline level, but this was not the case for the education alone group (Iwata and Becksfort, 1981). Providing an incentive was a more effective strategy than education alone.

Another study exploring the relative usefulness of various methods has been reported by Kegeles et al. (1978). All children were given a slide show about the aetiology of dental disease, health and cosmetic consequences of decay, and the effectiveness of fluoride as a preventive measure. They were then assigned to one of three groups. Those in one group were given no further attention, except that they were allowed to ask questions about the slide show. Those in the second group were given two discussion periods on the Health Belief Model, exploring ideas of seriousness, vulnerability and preventability (see Chapter 1 for a brief discussion of the Health Belief Model). The children in the third group were offered some small cash incentives if they volunteered for and continued through the treatment programme.

This treatment was then offered to all three groups. It involved using a mouthrinse at home twice a day from a bottle which contained a 14-day supply. The bottles were designed so that the children could not simply dispose of the contents all at once: a stopper ensured that they would be ready for use only at 6-hourly intervals. Every 2 weeks the bottles were to be returned, when the incentive group children were given a small reward, and the next bottle picked up. This procedure continued for 20 weeks. The results indicated that the information plus incentive condition was again the most effective, as shown in Fig. 2.1.

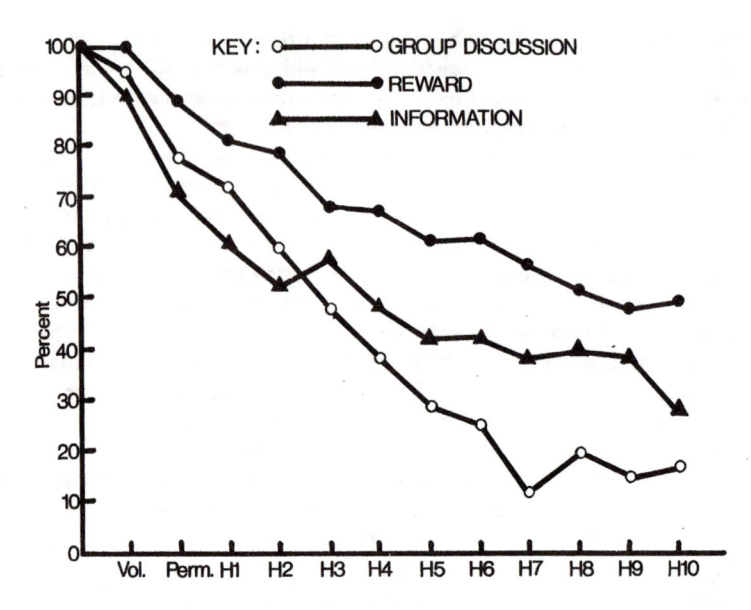

Figure 2.1 Percentages of children in each condition who complied with each stage of the mouthrinse programme. From Kegeles et al. (1978).

For example, 49% of the children given an incentive picked up the last bottle, 31% of the information only group and 18% of the discussion group children. That the discussion was the least effective is surprising but a similar result was found in another study in which the treatment involved topical fluoride applications (Lund et al., 1977).

Problems with material reinforcements

These studies are unsatisfactory for a number of reasons. While they illustrate that positive reinforcement is effective, they also show that it does not work for everyone. Only half the children in the study by Kegeles et al. completed the whole programme. This may be because the same reinforcement was offered to all children. Not everyone will be impressed by the same type of reward. Some patients may prefer cash, others toys and yet others badges. Another practical difficulty with these studies is that the cost of the rewards could add up to a considerable sum if a dentist were to offer them to all patients. The size of the reward may well be important since studies in other areas have shown that this is an important variable in changing behaviour. Generally, the smaller the reward the less likely it is that behaviour will be learned and maintained. There are several reports in the literature by dentists who use star systems. Patients are asked to keep a record card and every time a check-up is satisfactory a star is added to it. Bronze, silver or gold stars could be given, depending on the results.

Several dentists have claimed that such inexpensive rewards are useful, but a controlled study is required to evaluate the approach. The discussion of experimental design in this book may enable the practising dentist to conduct such studies with his or her own patients. The reader could give stars to one group of patients while providing the usual form of preventive care advice to another group. Over a period of 1 or 2 years, are there any differences in the amount of treatment required by each group? It would be important when testing for any differences that the measures of oral health were taken 'blind', i.e. by someone who did not know which patients had been given the reinforcements.

Many of these studies portray patients as passive recipients of reinforcements, seemingly being manipulated by the psychologists or dentists. This portrayal may not correspond particularly well to how we see ourselves or our relationships with patients. Nor do these studies involve parents, who are important in encouraging dental health habits in their children.

Involving parents in care
Every attempt should be made to encourage parental involvement when attempting to change a child's health habits. It is equally important that parents be helped to use positive reinforcement, rather than punishment, as illustrated by Claerhout and Lutzker (1981). They identified four children (5–9 years of age) who presented particular problems for their dentist because of their lack of regular oral health care at home. The children and the parents were invited to discuss the problem and the parents expressed their willingness to become involved. At first, the frequency of brushing was charted without reinforcements being given. Each time the children brushed a note was made on a calendar. This provided some baseline data, indicating to all concerned the exact nature of the problem. Snyder's test (which measures the amount of lactobacilli in the mouth) and Greene's index (for plaque) were also administered. Then, each time the children brushed twice per day at home they would be given a small reinforcement by their parents.

For two children simply placing stars on a calendar was sufficient to increase brushing from low baseline levels to almost 100% compliance. For the other two, small rewards were used: for example, once one child had gained 20 stars for regular care, some pocket money was given. The parents volunteered that they didn't mind giving cash reinforcements if this would help prevent serious future problems. An interesting aspect of this programme was that the children were involved in choosing their own reinforcements: in one case the child chose her own supper menu one day a week. This intervention increased brushing and had significant effects on lactobacilli and plaque scores. One year after the completion of the structured programme the parents of these children were again contacted and reported that the oral hygiene practices continued to be satisfactory.

Thumbsucking can also be reduced by such methods. It often occurs at times of stress (Lauterbach, 1990) and can be seen as a way in which children try to comfort themselves, so that sources of stress should be examined. However, De LaCruz and Geboy (1983) describe how they eliminated thumbsucking in an 8-year-old boy after various interventions had failed. The parents were asked to observe the child for an hour each day, charting the occasions when he was sucking his thumb. This indicated that he was thumbsucking about half the time. He was then told that if he could reduce his thumbsucking to about 25% of the time, he would be given a gold star for each day he accomplished this target. When he accumulated 7 stars, he would be able to choose an inexpensive gift.

Within 3 weeks thumbsucking was eliminated completely, including those times when receiving a gold star was not contingent on behaviour (e.g. when he was in bed). After 27 days, the child suggested termination of the programme himself, because the presence of the chart with the gold stars embarrassed him when friends visited and he no longer required it. Five months later, there was still no thumbsucking. A more thorough description of a similar procedure is given by Cripes et al. (1986).

Self-reinforcement
With adults, no externally provided reinforcements may be needed because they can be encouraged to reward themselves for performing health-care tasks. They are capable of choosing their own reinforcements (e.g. a new pair of shoes or a favourite meal) and administering them correctly. One variant of this is called the Premack principle. There are many actions in which people engage regularly—dressing in the morning, watering the house plants, watching television and so on. These kinds of behaviour can act as reinforcers for other kinds of behaviour if they are sequenced correctly. For example, patients could be asked not to dress in the morning until they have brushed their teeth, or not to watch television before flossing.

Modelling
People's behaviour depends not only on the consequences of their own actions but also on observing the consequences of others' behaviour. These observations provide valuable information about what can be expected from what behaviour. A dental student, for example, will learn much by watching how a qualified dentist goes about a restoration or talks with patients. If the restoration goes well, the student is likely to repeat the dentist's actions when practising him- or herself. If a student observes a dentist talking to a patient in a way which results in open and successful communication, he or she might later repeat such behaviour. On the other hand, if the patient becomes upset, the student may decide to treat patients differently. In other words, the teaching staff provide a model for the student, indicating which behaviour could be expected to have positive or negative consequences.

Modelling can have deleterious effects. One of the problems that medical educators have in changing smoking habits, for example, is that many smokers can cite examples of friends or relatives who smoked all their lives with few ill effects. Similarly, many people can cite examples of others who rarely visit the dentist yet seem to have healthy teeth and gums.

Modelling can also be used to change behaviour in more positive directions, as one study with dental students shows. Half the students from a class were given a dental examination and a plaque index was taken. They were then given intensive one-to-one training in oral hygiene and encouraged to follow the recommended procedures. Unexpectedly, 2 weeks later, plaque scores were again taken, this time for the whole class. As shown in Fig. 2.2 there was a great improvement for those given the training.

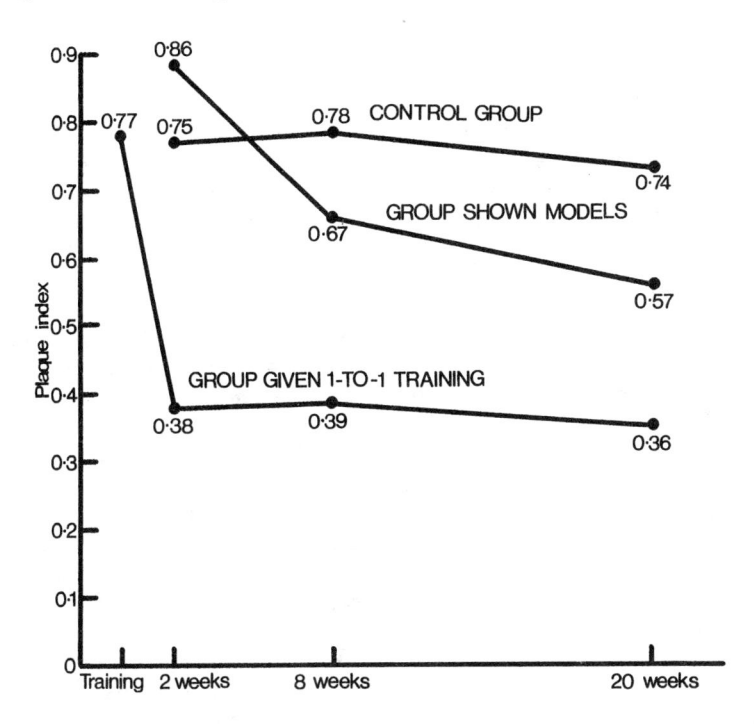

Figure 2.2 Changes in plaque index scores for students in each condition. Adapted from Newcombe (1974).

The results were then shown to the rest of the class while the students were highly praised for their improvement. The benefits of their behaviour were stressed. Thus, these students provided a model for good oral hygiene for the rest of the class. In order to test for the effectiveness of this modelling, the plaque scores for the whole class were again taken unexpectedly 6 weeks later and then again at 20 weeks. Figure 2.2 indicates that the group given the modelling showed a steady decrease in their plaque scores. It seems that people can be encouraged to improve their oral hygiene if they see others being rewarded for doing so and if they can see that improvement results from conscientious care (Newcombe, 1974).

Figure 2.2 also shows a control group of students who were not exposed to the modelling. This group was included to rule out two other possible interpretations of the results. It may have been the case that the students' plaque scores would improve over time anyway because during their course the benefits of brushing may have been stressed. Another possible reason for their improvement could have been that simply being examined called attention to plaque and this encouraged the students to brush and floss more conscientiously. By including this control group (who were dental students from another year), giving them dental examinations, and following their scores over time, these possibilities could be tested. Since the control group showed no improvement, these alternative interpretations of the results could be ruled out.

One distinct advantage of modelling is that it can be used in everyday dental practice. For example, when one child has a check-up which is satisfactory or better than the previous one, this could be rewarded in the presence of siblings. By seeing a brother or sister rewarded for good or improving hygiene, other members of a family may also be encouraged to take better care of their teeth and gums.

Highlighting negative consequences

Another possible method of increasing the likelihood of preventive care would be to provide negative reinforcements—those which increase the likelihood of behaviour when they are *removed*. In order for decay or extractions to be negatively reinforcing in themselves, it would be necessary for people to consider these possibilities as consequences to be avoided. However, this does not seem to be the case for many people. In one survey, only 10% of those interviewed thought that dental problems would have a significant effect on their jobs, appearance or social life. Many people also seem to expect that full dentures will not cause them problems, so that tooth loss is not considered to have negative consequences.

White (1980) described how he used negative reinforcement for encouraging his orthodontic patients to brush thoroughly. They were able to avoid having their teeth cleaned with a bitter-tasting preparation (quinine powder and flour of pumice) if they could clean their teeth well enough to remove plaque. Before the programme began about 12% of his patients had poor oral hygiene, but over the next 2 years this fell to 4%.

It can be argued that while this procedure seems to be effective (White's results would be more convincing if he included a control group) it raises some problems. Not the least of these is that many patients might well choose to change dentists rather than submit to such an experience. Instead of imposing negative consequences on patients, it might be sufficient to point out the results of poor dental care. Walsh et al. (1985) did this with some success by using gingival bleeding as a negative reinforcer. Patients who were taught that bleeding was a sign of disease and could be avoided by increased self-care showed a significant improvement in gingival health, a result which was not found for a control group of patients. Two further methods which have been used to heighten the salience of negative consequences are disclosing agents and arousing apprehension about the consequences of poor hygiene.

Disclosing agents

These are often used as part of educational programmes and for this reason it is difficult to disentangle their effects from other aspects of the packages. For example, in an experiment by Clark et al. (1973) children were presented with a traditional education programme on the problems which could be expected from poor dental hygiene. Information about how these problems could be overcome was given in two different ways. For half the children, instruction on flossing and brushing and the use of disclosing tablets was given in a lecture. Afterwards they were given a kit which included a supply of disclosing tablets and two toothbrushes. For the other half, the instruction was given personally. These children's teeth were stained and then examined for plaque by a dental hygienist and by other members of the group. Those showing plaque were given assistance in brushing and flossing. Furthermore, over the next 8 months, once a week, a dental assistant supervised the staining, flossing and brushing of teeth. Six months after the completion of the supervision all the children's teeth were again stained and measures taken. For the children in the group given the education programme alone, there was no change in the amount of debris on the teeth, but for those given specific and continuing instruction a highly significant reduction in plaque was found.

Some conclusions may be drawn from this study. Since both groups of children were given disclosing agents they alone could not have been responsible for the difference. Further, since there was no improvement for the first group, it seems unlikely that simply issuing disclosing tablets to patients will improve hygiene (although they may halt further deterioration—it was not possible to tell here without another control group). Other conclusions are more difficult to draw. Indeed, it is difficult to specify just what was responsible for the difference in plaque scores because there were several differences in procedure between the two groups. The students in the supervised group were instructed to examine each other's teeth, but this did not occur in the lecture-only group. The disclosing agent made plaque visible not only for the individual concerned but also for others. The condition of one's teeth became public knowledge. Perhaps it was this public disclosure which was important. It also seems probable that the dental hygienist was rewarding, through praise, those children whose plaque scores were improving. It may not have been the disclosing agent per se which was important, but rather the assistant's positive reactions to the state of the children's teeth.

Most studies which have supported the usefulness of disclosing agents have been similar to the one described, in that there have been several other components to the treatment package. Because of this, it is not possible to specify which variable or set of variables is responsible for any change. Disclosing agents do seem to be effective in informing patients about the state of their oral hygiene, particularly if photographs are used (Albino et al., 1977), but they may only be useful in changing behaviour if the plaque they show is considered to have some negative connotation. Simply issuing them to patients and hoping for the best is unlikely to be effective.

Arousing apprehension
A theme of this chapter is that people's behaviour is strongly influenced by its consequences. As suggested earlier, one reason why people do not

take better care of their teeth may be that they are unable to experience the negative consequences of neglect until it is too late. These consequences can be pointed out and this may account for at least some of the success of educational programmes. There remains the question of how these consequences should be portrayed. Would it be appropriate for a periodontist simply to state that poor oral hygiene can lead to tooth loss, or would a warning that edentulousness can be severely handicapping and distressing be more effective?

An influential study in this area was performed by Janis and Feshbach (1953), who were interested in the relative effectiveness of different levels of fear arousal. In their study three lectures were recorded, each of about the same length, each given by the same speaker in a standard manner, and each containing the same information about tooth decay and recommendations to avoid it. However, the lectures differed in the amount of fear they were designed to arouse. One lecture was accompanied by slides which vividly portrayed tooth decay and infections. It also emphasized the painful consequences of decay and diseased gums, reflecting the theory of focal infection which was popular at the time. For example, one passage included the warning:

> If you ever develop an infection of this kind from improper care of your teeth, it will be an extremely serious matter because these infections are really dangerous. They can spread to your eyes, or your heart, or your joints and cause secondary infections which may lead to diseases such as arthritic paralysis, kidney damage or total blindness (p. 79).

A second lecture described the same dangers in a more moderate and factual manner, using milder examples for the slides. The third lecture was designed to arouse minimal fear: diagrams and X-rays were used on the slides rather than photographs. The question was: which lecture would have the greatest effect on behaviour? It turned out to be the lecture designed to arouse minimal fear, where the negative consequences of neglect were explained but not vividly portrayed. The high fear arousal lecture actually seemed to have a deleterious effect on dental care.

There is an important corollary here, however. In another study (Haefner, 1965), using the same lecture material, the strong fear arousal lecture had the more positive effect on preventive care. Why this contradiction? It seemed that it had to do with the people in the study. Janis and Feshbach used children from well-to-do suburban homes in their research, while in the second study, most were from inner-city backgrounds. When the children in the second study were divided into upper- and lower-class groups, a striking difference was found. For the upper-class children the low fear arousal lecture was the most effective, while for the lower-class children the high fear arousal condition had the most effect.

In both these studies it is likely that education was an important part of the programme. As one child in the strong arousal condition of the Janis and Feshbach study volunteered: 'I don't think that you should have so many gory pictures without showing more to prevent it'. Arousing apprehension about the consequences of poor dental care seems useful, but it is also necessary to provide patients with ways of overcoming these possibilities. Sutton (1982) provides a review of the literature on fear arousal.

Punishment
Punishment is an unpleasant consequence which reduces the likelihood of behaviour being repeated. While punishment is effective in the short run, it seems to have few long-term effects: once the threat is no longer present, the behaviour often returns. There are also several problems with using punishment in a professional capacity. Not the least of these is ethical: does the dentist have the right to judge patients and their behaviour? The use of punishment has several connotations for patients, implying as it does that the dentist is in a position of power and authority over them. There may also be some doubt as to which behaviour will be reduced. For example, a patient may have a highly cariogenic diet because he or she sucks sugary mints throughout the day. Reprimanding the patient *may* curtail the consumption of mints, but conversely the patient may decide to change dentist to one who offers practical advice on non-cariogenic substitutes.

For these reasons, psychologists tend not to use punishment. Rather, they would look for instances of desirable behaviour and positively reinforce these. This was the method used with the young boy who was sucking his thumb, discussed earlier. Instead of reprimanding him when he was thumbsucking, his parents gave him reinforcements when he was not engaging in this behaviour. Similarly, if the aims were to change dietary habits, the procedure would be to praise the consumption of non-sugary foods rather than punish the eating of sweets. It is most likely that there will be some aspects of the patient's behaviour which are consistent with good oral health and these should be positively reinforced.

Individual differences

Personality

In many of the studies discussed in this chapter, the emphasis has been on behaviour and its environmental determinants rather than on what people think or believe about them. However this does not seem to be wholly adequate. In the study of Kegeles et al. (Fig. 2.1), for example, providing rewards for the children was more effective than providing information or encouraging discussion , yet only about half the children in the reward group completed the programme. Perhaps the rewards were not large enough or appropriate. Would the children have preferred badges or small toys? In any case, it is clear that there are individual differences in how people react to their environment. These differences can be attributed to personality variables and have formed an important aspect of psychological research.

Locus of control
A personality variable which has aroused considerable interest in the psychology of health care is known as *locus of control*. It refers to the

degree to which individuals perceive the events that happen to them as being contingent on their own behaviour or a result of external factors such as luck, chance or fate. Those who believe that they have control over what happens to them are termed 'internals' while those who believe that events are largely a matter of chance or fate are termed 'externals'. Thus, the belief has to do with contingency and consequence.

Locus of control is often measured using Rotter's (1966) scale. People are given several pairs of statements and asked to make a choice between them. For example, one pair is:

1 I have often found that what is going to happen will happen.
2 Trusting to fate has never turned out as well for me as making a decision to take a definite course of action.

The person is asked to choose the statement which most appropriately reflects his or her views. Those who tend to agree with statements which suggest that ability and effort are important (such as 2) would be internals, while those who believe that luck or fate determines what happens to them (such as 1) would be considered externals. Most people fall somewhere between the two extremes.

This concept has had considerable success when applied to preventive health care. As expected, internals, believing as they do that what happens to them is under their own control, take more preventive actions than do externals (see Strickland, 1978, for a review). Although two studies (Duke and Cohen, 1975; Kent et al., 1984) have found that locus of control scores are associated with preventive care and oral health, the conclusions must be tentative since some other studies have shown no effect. This might be because the Rotter scale is not sufficiently subtle. More recently, it has been pointed out that someone who has an external locus of control could believe either that oral health is largely a matter of chance (i.e. is essentially uncontrollable by anyone) or that oral health can be influenced by someone else, such as a professional (i.e. that it is controllable, but not by patients themselves). Thus the external dimension can be subdivided into two scales: one to do with the belief that health cannot be controlled by anyone, the other to do with the belief that a professional can influence health.

When Galgut et al. (1986) gave this modified version of locus of control to patients, they found that those with high scores on the internal dimension as well as the external professional care dimension responded favourably to oral hygiene instruction (as measured by lower levels of plaque and gingivitis), but those who believed that oral health was largely a matter of chance did not benefit from instruction.

Thus, it is possible to see how different patients may need to be managed in different ways. Those who believe that oral health is largely a matter of chance may require external reinforcements to encourage them to be conscientious in appointment-keeping and regular home care. Small rewards might be offered to them or the negative consequences of poor oral hygiene stressed. Those who believe that professional care is needed may be more likely to accept advice and attend appointments for oral health screening. Internals on the other hand might be left alone, once the contingencies have been pointed out, to monitor themselves. The advantage of such a categorization of patients is that the dentist would be able to predict which patients are likely to present management problems, rather than waiting to see which are unco-operative or miss appointments. Just how accurately a dentist could ascertain an individual's locus of control without the rather obtrusive measure of using a personality questionnaire is open to question and remains to be tested.

Designing a preventive programme

It must be said at the outset that a dentist who hopes to make large and clinically significant changes in most patients' behaviour is likely to be disappointed. It is very difficult to accomplish this in the few minutes a year which is available for most patients. This is partly because oral health will not have the same priority for most patients as it will for a dentist, and partly because it is difficult to change habitual patterns of behaviour. In one survey, over 40% of adults said that they had not changed their hygiene habits at all after being given instructions by their dentists. Nevertheless, over 50% of the sample claimed that they did make some changes, even if they were minimal. Some changed to a particular toothbrush design, for example. The challenge of preventive dentistry is to increase the likelihood of change and to ensure that it is maintained in the future.

In applying the principles of contingency and reinforcement explained in this chapter, there are several ground rules which must be followed if they are to be effective. Most of the six steps outlined below have been discussed previously, but this section provides a working summary which could be useful for the practising dentist. Each patient will require a slightly different approach since for each individual there will be a unique set of circumstances and problems.

1 A clear and precise definition of the problem

Many people are unaware of the basic facts and do not have the skills needed for adequate prevention. As discussed earlier, it is important that verbal advice is supplemented by written material whenever possible. It is equally important that patients should be able to understand and remember this information. A rather detailed assessment may be needed so that gaps in knowledge and skills may be identified and filled.

However, this will not be sufficient for all patients. The information may not be put into practice. In such a case the problem can be seen in terms of antecedents and consequences. In order to change behaviour, it is important to specify exactly what requires alteration. To say that the patient has 'poor dental health' is not adequate, since this is too global and vague a definition and could be due to many different factors. More specific *behavioural* definitions are needed since patients must know which of their health care patterns must be changed. A thorough inspection of the patient's oral cavity will highlight the major health problem.

For example, if the patient has severe gingivitis, this suggests that brushing and flossing must be improved. The presence of new carious lesions indicates the consumption of many cariogenic snacks and drinks, so diet needs attention.

2 Monitoring the frequency of the problem behaviour

Once the broad nature of the specific difficulty is identified, it is important to gain some information about current behaviour. This can be achieved by charting the incidence of a particular behaviour. This serves three purposes. First, it provides both the patient and the dentist with some information about the scope of the problem. This helps to define it. Second, the patient is able to see that he or she is making progress in attempts to change behaviour. This can have beneficial effects in itself. Third, charting provides the dentist with a way of monitoring the effectiveness of the preventive programme. Although it is unlikely that the chart will be completely accurate, if a baseline is gathered before an intervention begins progress can be checked.

To give a practical example: a patient visits the dentist with several cavities which will require several appointments to restore. The problem seems to be that the patient consumes cariogenic foods at frequent intervals throughout the day. In order to gauge the exact frequency of this behaviour, the patient could be asked to place a tick on a prepared sheet each time sugar is eaten. The range of foods which contain sugar would need to be explained. The patient might also be asked to indicate the circumstances in which this occurs—the antecedents. Over a period of 1 or 2 weeks before the next appointment the patient will be able to see—and perhaps be surprised at—the amount and timing of sugar consumption. It may be more effective if the dentist provides a chart rather than leaving it to the patient. An example is shown in Table 2.1.

Table 2.1 An example of a chart which could be used to monitor the frequency and circumstances of eating sugary foods. The patient indicates whenever a sugary snack is eaten. In order to find out what triggers this behaviour, the circumstances (e.g. during morning coffee break) are also noted

Time	Date	Circumstances
8.00–9.00		
9.00–10.00		
10.00–11.00		
11.00–12.00		
12.00–1.00		
.		
.		
.		

3 Specifying the aims of the intervention

Just as it is important to specify the nature of the problem, so too is it important to consider what the dentist and patient aim to achieve. This is called the *target* behaviour. For a patient who eats five sugary snacks a day, the aim might be to reduce this to one per day. For someone who never flosses, the aim might be to floss thoroughly twice a week at specific times.

4 Changing the behaviour

However, these overall targets may not be easily achieved. Research has shown that it is very difficult to change patients' habits. Requesting a patient to make an abrupt and extensive change in diet, for example, is unlikely to have any effect. But it does seem possible to change small aspects of behaviour one at a time, so that over a long period considerable changes can be made. By taking realistically small steps, which the patient can reasonably be expected to achieve, the ultimate goal can be reached.

Shaping
The procedure which is used to accomplish this is called *shaping*. Horner and Keilitz (1975) describe how they used shaping in order to teach patients with severe intellectual handicaps to brush their teeth. While brushing is relatively easy for most people, it involves a complex series of behaviours which can be a formidable task for mentally handicapped people. In shaping, the steps needed in order to attain a final goal are noted. Then each of these steps, in turn, is reinforced until the whole series is learned.

In order to ascertain exactly what behaviours are involved in toothbrushing, Horner and Keilitz first videotaped a competent person brushing his teeth. From this tape they identified several small steps:

1 Pick up and hold the toothbrush.
2 Wet the toothbrush.
3 Remove cap of toothpaste.
4 Apply toothpaste to brush.
5 Replace cap on the toothpaste.
Steps 6–11 involve brushing various parts of the mouth
12 Rinse the toothbrush.
13 Rinse the sink.
14 Put equipment away.
15 Discard any paper cups or tissue used.

The teaching of each of these steps was accomplished by giving rewards. When the mentally handicapped patient picked up and held the toothbrush, for example, he was praised or given tokens which could be exchanged for sugarless gum. When this learning was accomplished, the next step was taught: rewards were given only when the toothbrush was wetted. These two pieces of behaviour were then *chained* together so that a reward was given only when the patient both picked up the toothbrush and wetted it. Then the next step was taught. This procedure was followed until the whole series of actions could be accomplished. Brushing one's teeth might form only a small part of an overall programme of self-care which could also include such skills as dressing, eating with utensils and so on.

Brushing
A similar procedure of rewarding small pieces of behaviour, one at a time, can be used for teaching children to brush their teeth. Accepted wisdom has it that children do not have the necessary motor skills to brush their teeth adequately until they are 7 or 8 years of age, but some research (Poche et al., 1982), suggests that children between 3 and 4 years of age can learn to brush competently. In their study toothbrushing was broken down into 16 steps, representing the cleaning of different parts of the mouth. At each step the children were required to hold the brush at a 45° angle and to use a soft scrubbing motion. Before training, the children were able to perform only about 9% of the necessary actions, but afterwards they were able to accomplish 96% of the necessary actions. At an 8-week follow-up, 87% of the steps were performed. This increased ability also resulted in a decrease in plaque levels. Thus, this study suggests that young children do have the necessary motor skills but that they may require more detailed training than older children.

Dietary changes
Similarly, diet can be altered. The aim would be to reduce sugar intake *slowly*. If, at baseline, the patient was having five cariogenic snacks per day, the first step might be to cut this down to four. When this has been accomplished, some reinforcement would be given and the next step would be to reduce this to three, and so on. During this time the patient would continue to chart eating habits and bring the charts to each dental appointment. At the same time an alternative behaviour could be encouraged: instead of eating sugary foods, sugarless gum could be substituted. The frequency of this behaviour would also be monitored and reinforced.

5 Reinforcement

The consequences of any change in behaviour should always be made clear. There is the praise and encouragement of the dentist but, as mentioned earlier in the chapter, most people are quite capable of reinforcing themselves. Once a certain level of sugar intake has been achieved, the patients could reinforce themselves with a new coat or a day-trip somewhere—whatever they find rewarding. Over the next few weeks, a lower sugar intake would be required before the reinforcement was given, and so on.

Reinforcements should be provided as soon as possible after the desired behaviour. In part, simply marking a chart or calendar serves this purpose, since the patient can see some positive consequence of the behaviour. This feedback can itself be useful encouragement. Immediate reinforcement is particularly important for children, who will be less likely than adults to appreciate a link between brushing on Monday and a trip to see a film on Saturday. Here the involvement of parents is crucial since only they are in a position to dispense a reinforcement immediately after brushing. The frequency with which reinforcements are given should decrease as time goes on, particularly after the target behaviour is reached. The ultimate aim is to integrate oral health habits within the patient's everyday activities so that they become habitual.

6 Failures in preventive programmes

It would be misleading to suggest that the kind of approach advocated in this chapter would be helpful to all patients and for this reason it is important for the dentist to monitor a patient's progress. There are several reasons why such a programme could fail. Perhaps the chosen reinforcement is not appropriate or sufficiently enticing, or perhaps the patient is not comfortable with rewarding him- or herself: further encouragement may be required. Another possibility concerns lack of support from parent or spouse. Programmes where other members of the family are involved typically have much higher success rates than those which concentrate solely on the patient.

Motivation
Motivation might be a problem. Weinstein et al. (1983) argue that 'When the patient does not desire to change, or does not perceive that a problem worth acting on exists, there is little a practitioner can do' (p. 68). Motivation can be increased by asking the patient to make a list of the reasons why the behaviour should change. Stressing the importance of physical appearance or the lowered chances of tooth loss might be very useful in this respect.

A related problem is that of commitment. Although a patient may indicate that he or she intends to follow a programme, these good intentions may not be translated into behaviour. One method for increasing commitment is termed 'contracting'. Although it may seem rather artificial, it has proved an effective approach. The patient is asked to sign a form, such as that shown in Table 2.2, which is a 'public' commitment to the programme. In some studies patients have been asked to deposit a sum of money which would be returned only if they complete the programme—an especially successful method.

Table 2.2 A possible contract for monitoring sugar consumption

Before my next appointment on_____
I agree to:
1 Carry the chart with me whenever I am likely to eat a snack.
2 Tick the chart each time I eat a snack containing sugar.
3 Consider what it could be doing to my teeth.
4 Bring the chart to my next appointment.

Signed_____ Date_____

The staff's role

Other reasons why a preventive programme might not succeed concerns the views of staff. There are two possibilities here. One is that the dentist or other staff might have reservations about implementing the programme consistently and enthusiastically. It may seem that the patient is being manipulated in some way. This is not the aim. Rather, it is to maximize the probability that patients will engage in dental health behaviours and find the consequences of this behaviour rewarding. The staff's role is to instigate and support the programme, but the final responsibility for its effectiveness is the patient's. Since staff are unlikely to be able to discuss dental problems with a patient for more than a few minutes per year, it is important that the maximum benefit should be gained from these interviews.

The other possibility is that the programme is instituted mechanically, without due concern for the interpersonal aspects of the situation. As discussed in Chapter 7, how staff relate to patients is often more important than what they advise. While information is of course necessary, it may well be less critical than patients' feelings that they are being cared for and understood.

The social context

Another possible reason why a preventive programme may fail is the patient's social context. There may be a lack of support from a spouse or parent. Although every patient's social context needs to be taken into account, perhaps the most problematic is the child's social world. Cariogenic foods are very important for children, not simply because they are inherently pleasant to eat, but also because they form part of the social system of exchange. The sharing of sugary foods provides an important means of reaffirming friendships and gaining status. From a child's point of view, the everyday contingencies of the playground may be much more compelling than those of the occasional visit to the dentist. The replacement of non-cariogenic foods may be possible, but the cost to the child must be considered.

Summary

One reason why many people neglect their oral health may be a lack of knowledge and skills. Educational programmes have had little direct effect on oral health because the information is not always put into use. This could occur because the contingencies between controlling sugar consumption and brushing on the one hand and caries and gingival disease on the other are not obvious. Several methods can be used to improve home care. One possibility is providing positive reinforcement, either directly through inexpensive rewards or indirectly through modelling. Other members of the family can be involved in such programmes and patients can be shown how to monitor and reinforce their own behaviour. The aim is to integrate new patterns of dental care within the habitual routines of everyday life. People can also be helped to appreciate and avoid the negative consequences of neglect. Whatever the method used, it is important that the required changes are specified very clearly and precisely and that these changes are made slowly in small and realistic steps.

Practice implications

1 Dental practitioners are in a good position to remedy any lack of knowledge but it is important to make individual assessments and tailor information according to ability to understand.
2 Written information is a useful memory aid.
3 When attempting to change behaviour use positive reinforcements rather than reprimands.
4 Changing habits is difficult and time-consuming. Don't try to do too much at once and accept that, despite your best efforts, it will be possible to change the behaviour of only a minority of patients.

Suggested reading

For a more thorough discussion of psychological principles applied to transmitting information, see Ley P. *Communicating with Patients* (London, Croom Helm, 1988) and for preventive dental care, see Weinstein P., Getz T. *Changing Human Behaviour: Strategies for Preventive Dentistry* (London, Mosby, 1978).

References

Albino J. E., Julian D. B., Slakter M. J. (1977) Effects of an instructional programme on plaque and gingivitis in adolescents. *J. Public Health Dent.* **37**, 281–9.

Blinkhorn A. S. (1978) Influence of social norms on toothbrushing behaviour of pre-school children. *Community Dent. Oral Epidemiol.* 6, 222–6.

Blinkhorn A.S., Verity J.M. (1979) Assessment of the readability of dental health education literature. *Community Dent. Oral Epidemiol.* **7**,195–8.

Cripes M.H., Miraglia M., Gaulin-Kremer E.G. (1986) Monitoring and reinforcement to eliminate thumbsucking *J. Dent. Child.* **53**,48–52.

Claerhout S., Lutzker J. R. (1981) Increasing children's self-initiated compliance to dental regimes. *Behav. Ther.* **12**, 165–76.

Clark C. A., Fintz J. B., Elwell K. R. (1973) Eliminating dental plaque in the sixth grade. *J. Public Health Dent.* **33**, 70–4.

Craft M., Croucher R. (1980) *The 16 to 20 Study*. London: Health Education Council.

De LaCruz M., Geboy M. J. (1983) Elimination of thumbsucking through contingency management. *J. Dent. Child.* **50**, 39–41.

Duke M. P., Cohen B. (1975) Locus of control as an indicator of patient cooperation. *J. Am. Coll. Dent.* **42**, 174–8.

Flesch R.P. (1951) *How to Test Readability*. New York: Harper & Row.

Galgut P.N., Waite I.M., Todd-Pokropek A., Barnby G.J. (1986) The relationship between the multidimensional health locus of control and the performance of subjects on a preventive periodontal programme. *J. Clin. Periodontol.* **14**,171–5.

Haefner D. P. (1965) Arousing fear in dental health education. *J. Public Health Dent.* **25**, 140–6.

Horner R. D., Keilitz I. (1975) Training mentally retarded adolescents to brush their teeth. *J. Appl. Behav. Anal.* **8**, 301–9.
Horowitz A. M., Suomi J. D., Peterson J. K. et al. (1976) Effects of supervised daily dental plaque removal by children. *J. Public Health Dent.* **36**, 193–200.
Iwata B. A., Becksfort C. M. (1981) Behavioural research in preventive dentistry. *J. Appl. Behav. Anal.* **14**, 111–20.
Janis I. L., Feshbach S. (1953). Effects of fear-arousing communication. *J. Abnorm. Soc. Psychol.* **48**, 78–92.
Kanouse D.E., Hayes-Roth B. (1980) Cognitive considerations in the design of product warnings. In *Banbury Report 6: Product Labelling and Health Risks* (Morris L.A., Mazzio M., Barofsky I., eds). Cold Spring Harbor: Cold Spring Harbor Laboratories.
Kegeles S. S., Lund A. K., Weisenberg M. (1978) Acceptance by children of a daily home mouthrinse programme. *Soc. Sci. Med.* **12**, 199–210.
Kent G., Matthews R., White F. (1984) Locus of control and oral health. *J. Am. Dent. Assoc.* **109**, 67–9.
Lauterbach W. (1990) Stimulus-response (S-R) questions for identifying the function of problem behaviour: the example of thumb sucking. *Br. J. Clin. Psychol.* **29**, 51–7.
Levine B.A., Moss K.C., Ramsey P.H. et al. (1978) Patient compliance with advice as a function of communicator expertise. *J. Soc. Psychol.* **104**, 309–10.
Ley P. (1988) *Communicating with Patients.* London: Croom Helm.
Linn E.L. (1974) What dental patients don't know about dental care. *J. Public Health Dent.* **34**, 39–41.
Lund A. K., Kegeles S. S., Weisenberg M. (1977) Motivational techniques for increasing acceptance of preventive health measures. *Med. Care* **15**, 678–92.
Martens L. U., Frazier P. J., Kirt K. J. et al. (1973) Developing brushing performance in second graders through behaviour modification. *Health Serv. Rep.* **88**, 818–23.
Newcombe G. M. (1974) Instruction in oral hygiene for a group of dental students: its effects on their peers. *J. Public Health Dent.* **34**, 113–16.
Poche C., McCubbrey H., Munn T. (1982) The development of correct toothbrushing technique. *J. Appl. Behav. Anal.* **15**, 315–20.
Poulton E.C., Warren T., Bond J. (1970) Ergonomics in journal design. *Appl. Ergonomics* **13**, 207–9.
Reiss M. L., Piotrowski W. D., Bailey J. S. (1976) Behavioural community psychology: encouraging low income parents to seek dental care for their children. *J. Appl. Behav. Anal.* **9**, 387–97.
Rotter J. B. (1966) Generalized expectancies for internal versus external locus of control of reinforcement. *Psychol. Monogr.* **80**, 1–28.
Strickland B. R. (1978) Internal-external expectancies and health-related behaviour. *J. Consult. Clin. Psychol.* **46**, 1192–211.
Sutton S.R. (1982) Fear arousing communications: a critical examination of research and theory. In *Social Psychology and Behavioural Medicine.* (J.R. Eiser, ed.). New York: Wiley.
Todd, J.E., Walker, A., Dodd, P. (1982) *Adult Dental Health vol. 2. United Kingdom, 1978.* London: HMSO.
Walsh M.M., Heckman B.H., Moreau-Diettinger R. (1985) Use of gingival bleeding for reinforcement of oral home care behaviour. *Community Dent. Oral Epidemiol.* **13**, 133–5.
Weinstein P., Getz, T.and Milgrom, R. (1983). Oral self-care: a promising alternative behavior model. *J. Am. Dent. Assoc.* **107**, 67–70.
White L. W. (1980) Behaviouristic technique for oral hygiene: an update. *Am. J. Orthodont.* **77**, 568–70.
Zifferblat S. M. (1975) Increasing patient compliance through the applied analysis of behaviour. *Prevent. Med.* **4**, 173–82.

Chapter 3

The nature and causes of anxiety

Anxiety experienced by dental patients is of concern, partly because of its effects on patients and partly because of its effects on dentists themselves. There seems little doubt that patients' anxiety can interfere with dental care. Surveys typically show that a sizeable proportion of the general population avoid making regular visits to the dentist because they are too frightened to do so. In a survey of 6000 people, 43% reported that they avoided going to the dentist unless they were experiencing trouble with their teeth (Todd and Walker, 1980). Of these, 58% said that part of the reason was that they were 'scared of the dentist' (Todd et al., 1982). Further evidence that anxiety contributes to delay in visiting the dentist is provided by Curson and Coplans (1970). When they interviewed 100 patients in an emergency clinic, 38% said that they did not make regular visits because they were too afraid of the experience. Of these, only 12% made and kept further appointments for a course of treatment.

Such results have several implications for the dental practitioner. On the one hand, they mean that dentists will encounter some patients who require extensive restorative work yet will not agree to have it. On the other hand, the anxious patient can present personal and interpersonal problems. As mentioned in Chapter 1, a survey of stresses encountered by dentists indicated that the most important problem was 'coping with difficult patients', many of whom are anxious. For the dentist who considers himself or herself as someone who wishes to help patients and improve their quality of life, it can be disturbing to be seen as someone who inflicts distress. The first section of this chapter considers a view of anxiety that is shared by many psychologists. This outline of the nature of anxiety is useful in understanding its aetiology, a topic discussed in the second half of the chapter. The practical significance of this research is discussed in Chapter 4, where methods of alleviating anxiety are considered.

The nature of anxiety

Many definitions of anxiety have been suggested, sometimes resulting in confusion when the word is used in different ways. For a psychoanalyst, anxiety refers to a result of a complex interplay between various parts of the personality. It is beyond the scope of this book to discuss the psychoanalytic viewpoint, although the reader may find a paper by Lewis (1957) an interesting introduction. Amongst psychologists, the term 'anxiety' has been used in several ways. For some, anxiety is a 'vague, unpleasant feeling accompanied by a premonition that something undesirable is about to happen' (Kagan and Havemann, 1976). This is primarily a subjective definition, relying on how people feel. Other psychologists prefer to use a behavioural definition, arguing that the presence of anxiety is best indicated by how a person acts. This could be measured by whether a patient avoids visiting the dentist or is reluctant to let the dentist use instruments. Sometimes a distinction is made between anxiety and fear: anxiety is said to be a general feeling of discomfort while fear is considered to be a reaction to a specific event or object. For example, a person might be anxious about a visit to the dentist and specifically fearful about an extraction. Often the words anxiety and fear are used interchangeably, however, and no distinction will be made here.

This lack of agreement about how to define anxiety means that it has been measured in different ways. In the studies discussed in this chapter, subjective, behavioural and physiological measures have been used. On a behavioural measure of avoidance, for example, a patient who attends a dentist regularly might not be considered anxious, yet if he or she expresses worry or concern it would seem inappropriate to classify this person as non-anxious. Conversely, someone may refuse to see a dentist yet deny any suggestion of anxiety. Rather than debate which kind of measure is the more valid, in recent years psychologists have tended to consider all of them important, reflecting different aspects of the problem. Seen in this way, anxiety can be broken down into a number of constituent variables, each making a contribution to our understanding. Some researchers have examined how different situations evoke anxiety, others have concentrated on subjective reports while yet others have explored physiological and behavioural components.

The situation

Intuitively, some situations are more anxiety-provoking than others. Agras et al. (1969) found that in the USA visiting the dentist ranked fourth, behind snakes, heights and storms. Some people have inordinately intense fears of particular situations, so much so that they will avoid contact at almost any cost. Such intense fears, called phobias, seem to be out of all proportion to the actual threat and do not respond to reason. The potential effects of such fears has been illustrated by Lautch (1971) who found that phobic patients suffered pain for an average 17.3 days before consulting a dentist, as compared to only 3.0 days for a matched sample of non-phobics. Such suffering is not uncommon: Segal (1986) reported that 15% of the patients attending an emergency clinic had been in pain for 1 month or more.

Sources of anxiety
It would be useful to specify which dental procedures are associated with the most anxiety. Wardle (1982a) asked patients attending a dental

Table 3.1 Ranking of dental situations from the most feared to the least feared for high-fear and low-fear groups

Situation	Low-fear group	High-fear group
Dentist is pulling your tooth	1	2
Dentist is drilling your tooth	2	1
Dentist tells you that you have bad teeth	3	3
Dentist holds the syringe and needle in front of you	4	6
Dentist is giving you a shot	5	4
Have a probe placed in a cavity	6	5
Dentist laughs as he looks in your mouth	7	10
Dentist squirts air into a cavity	8	7
Sitting in the dentist's waiting room	9	8
Dentist is laying out his instruments	10	13
Nurse tells you it is your turn	12	9
Getting in the dentist's chair	11	11
Dentist is putting in the filling	13	14
Thinking about going to the dentist	15	12
Dentist cleans your teeth with steel probe	14	16
Getting in your car to go to the dentist	16	15
Dentist looks at your chart	17	17
Dentist places cotton in your mouth	18	18
Calling a dentist to make an appointment	19	19
Dental assistant places a bib on you	20	20
Dentist squirts water in your mouth	21	22
Making another appointment with the nurse	22	21
Dentist is cleaning your teeth	23	23
Dentist asks you to rinse your mouth	24	24
Dentist tells you he is through	25	25

From Gale (1972), with permission.

hospital to rate how anxious they would feel if they had to undergo each of a list of procedures. The patients were asked to indicate if they would be not anxious, slightly anxious, fairly anxious, very anxious or extremely anxious for each procedure. Extraction led the list, followed by injection and drilling. Polishing was the least feared. Similar results have been found with other groups, as shown in Table 3.1 (Gale, 1972). Here, a longer list of procedures is given but the general order is similar to Wardle's results.

Table 3.1 makes another important point, however: the amount of fear that a person experiences cannot be specified from knowledge of the situation alone. The patients were divided into high- and low-fear groups according to their overall feelings about visiting the dentist. The rankings of the procedures for the two groups were virtually identical (a correlation of 0.98 where a perfect correlation would equal 1.0). Although there was much agreement about the relative stressfulness of the various procedures, there were also important individual differences in the amount of anxiety each one provoked.

All of the people involved in these studies were dental patients. Do other people see the problems in the same way? Jackson (1978) gave a longer list of 60 items to several different groups—dentists, hygienists, dental students, dental patients and dental phobics—and asked them to rank the items for their stressfulness. Some items were ranked higher than others for all groups: 'Dentist is giving you a shot' and 'Having a root canal done' are two examples of high-stress items. However, there were some important differences in how the various groups ranked the items overall. Patients said that 'Dentist squirts water into your mouth' and 'Dentist prepares a shot of Novocain' were more stressful than did the dentists and hygienists. A particularly interesting finding concerned the rankings of the dental phobics: they found anticipating the dental visit (e.g. 'Getting into your car to go to the dentist' and 'Sitting in the dentist's waiting room') more stressful than did most of the other groups.

Another indication that it is not necessarily the drilling and filling which patients find frightening comes from the survey mentioned at the beginning of the chapter (Todd et al., 1982) which included edentulous patients. They have nothing to fear in these ways, yet 37% said that they sometimes delayed visiting because they were scared of the dentist.

These findings indicate that the amount of fear a person experiences cannot be specified from knowledge of the treatment alone. Although there is much agreement between patients about the relative stressfulness of various procedures, there are also important individual differences in the amount of fear each one provokes. Thus it is important and useful to have standard ways of measuring how anxious each individual feels.

Self-reports of anxiety

There are several questionnaires available which can be used to measure the amount of anxiety a person experiences. Some of these can be used in a variety of situations. The same questionnaire could be used whether the person is about to see a dentist, to take a university examination or to make a parachute jump. Other questionnaires are specific to certain settings in that they ask people how they feel about particular experiences, such as surgery or dentistry.

A general measure of anxiety
One popular method of measuring anxiety which can be used in many settings is the State–Trait Anxiety Inventory (STAI) developed by Speilberger (Speilberger et al., 1983). They make a distinction between anxiety as a general personality trait and anxiety as a response to a particular situation. The former is known as *trait anxiety*. People with high trait anxiety are those whose feelings of personal adequacy and worth are threatened by a wide variety of circumstances, particularly where some kind of failure is a possibility. *State anxiety*, by contrast, is more transitory, depending not so much on stable personality characteristics as on the specific situation. This type of anxiety varies as a function of the stresses which impinge on the person at a particular time. High state anxiety is evoked when an individual perceives a situation as threatening to physical or emotional well-being.

The STAI consists of 40 statements: 20 are designed to measure trait anxiety, while the other 20 measure state anxiety. An example of a trait item is 'I lack self-confidence' and the individual chooses one of four alternatives (almost never, sometimes, often or almost always) which best describes his or her feelings. In measuring state anxiety, the individual is asked to respond according to how he or she feels at the moment. For example, the item 'I feel calm' could be given one of the following four responses: not at all, somewhat, moderately so or very much so.

The STAI has been used extensively in dental research. Measures of state anxiety are particularly informative. Scores on these items of the STAI typically rise before a visit and then fall sharply afterwards. As discussed in the next chapter, state anxiety can be altered considerably with short-term minimal interventions. The measurement of trait anxiety can also be informative. Wardle (1982a) gave her patients the trait anxiety items from the STAI while they were waiting for treatment at a dental hospital. She also asked them how anxious they currently felt, how long it had been since their last visit, and took a number of physiological measures. No association was found between trait anxiety and current subjective feelings of anxiety or between trait anxiety and time since their last visit, but she did find a significant relationship with the number of signs of physiological arousal the patients were experiencing, such as sweatiness of the hands and dryness of the mouth.

Measuring dental anxiety

Besides questionnaires such as the STAI which can be used in many situations, there are several questionnaires which have been specifically designed to measure anxiety in the dental setting. In order to arrive at the rankings shown in Table 3.1, patients were asked to indicate on a 7-point scale between 'no fear' and 'terror' their degree of fear about each of the procedures mentioned.

Another questionnaire is the Dental Anxiety Scale (DAS) developed by Corah (1969). This is shown in Table 3.2. Patients are asked to circle the alternative which best represents how they feel. Each alternative is given a simple numerical value from 1 to 5 so that a total score could

Table 3.2 The Dental Anxiety Scale

1 If you had to go to the dentist tomorrow, how would you feel about it?
  a I would look forward to it as a reasonably enjoyable experience.
  b I wouldn't care one way or the other.
  c I would be a little uneasy about it.
  d I would be afraid that it would be unpleasant and painful.
  e I would be very frightened of what the dentist might do.
2 When you are waiting in the dentist's office for your turn in the chair, how do you feel?
  a Relaxed.
  b A little uneasy.
  c Tense.
  d Anxious.
  e So anxious that I sometimes break out in a sweat or almost feel physically sick.
3 When you are in the dentist's chair waiting while he gets his drill ready to begin working on your teeth, how do you feel? (Same alternatives as number 2.)
4 You are in the dentist's chair to have your teeth cleaned. While you are waiting and the dentist is getting out the instruments which he will use to scrape your teeth around the gums, how do you feel? (Same alternatives as number 2.)

From Corah (1969), with permission.

range from 4 to 20. A score of 13–14 should alert the dentist and patients with a score of 15 or more are almost always highly anxious (Corah et al., 1978).

Kleinknecht et al. (1973) have developed another approach, asking patients about their anxieties about a total of 27 specific items, such as making an appointment, seeing the needle and hearing the drill. Patients are asked to rate their fearfulness on a 1–5 scale, from 'none' to 'great' for each situation. This method provides a more precise view of a patient's anxiety than does Corah's DAS, giving detailed information which might be useful when attempting to alleviate the problem. These

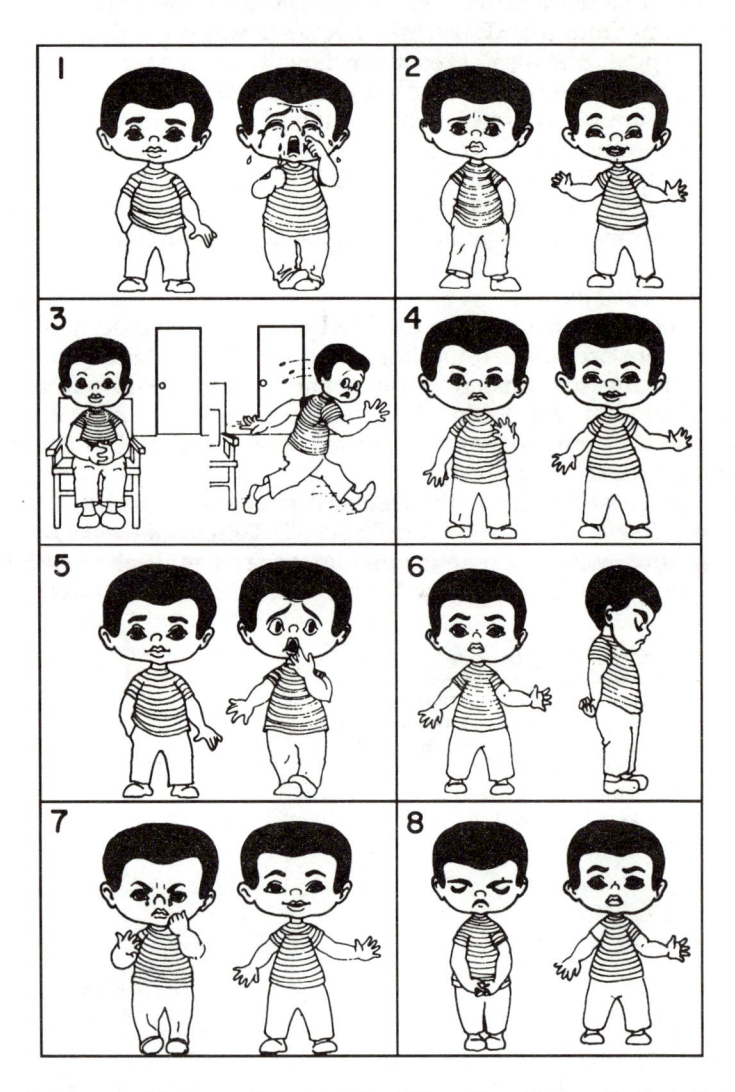

Figure 3.1 A method for assessing anxiety in children. The child is asked to indicate which drawing from each pair best describes how he or she feels. From Venham (1979) with permission.

researchers have, however, found that responses to one question ('Generally, how fearful are you of dentistry?') correlate 0.89 with responses to all the other items (Kleinknecht and Bernstein, 1978), suggesting that this might be a useful question for preliminary screening of patients.

A method for assessing anxiety in children is shown in Fig. 3.1. Venham (1979) asked the children in his study to choose which of the two alternatives on each of the eight cards best represented how they felt. A measure of anxiety was provided by totalling the number of times the child picked the cartoon depicting distress of some kind.

Validity of questionnaires
Instruments which aim to measure anxiety (or indeed any psychological factor, such as personality) must fulfil certain conditions. An important requirement is that they can be shown to be valid, i.e. they must measure what they purport to measure. This can be shown in several ways. For example, scores on the state anxiety items of the STAI would be expected to be different before and after a person undergoes a stressful experience. This has been done in a study on dental patients (Tullman et al., 1979). All were attending the dentist on a regular basis but one group was due to have only a check-up while the other group was scheduled for some treatment, such as a restoration. While they were waiting to see the dentist, all patients were given the state anxiety questionnaire to complete. As expected, the patients waiting for restorations reported higher anxiety than those waiting for their check-up. When given the questionnaire at the completion of the appointment, the treatment patients showed a significant decrease. At this point the anxiety reported by the two groups was similar. These results show that the STAI state anxiety scale is sensitive to differences in the situation.

Another method of validating self-report questionnaires is to take physiological and behavioural measures and relate these to subjective feelings. People who have a high pulse rate at the dental surgery or who avoid attending whenever possible should score higher on self-report measures than those whose pulse is slower or who make regular visits. Corah used dentists' ratings of patient anxiety to validate his DAS. He first asked patients to fill out the questionnaire and then asked dentists to rate the patients' anxiety without knowing their responses on the scale. He found a significant relationship between these scores, indicating some validity.

Reliability of questionnaires
It is also important to investigate the reliability of these questionnaires. Reliability is tested by asking the same group of people to fill out the questionnaire on two occasions, some months apart. If very different answers were given at these two times, it would mean that the questionnaire was measuring a transitory feeling rather than longer-term anxiety. When Corah did this on the DAS at a 3-month interval he found a good correlation between the two scores ($r = 0.82$), indicating that the reliability of this questionnaire is high.

Most of the questionnaires mentioned here have been shown to have adequate validity and reliability. This means that they can be used with some confidence by a researcher or a dentist who wishes to measure subjective anxiety. It also means that the effectiveness of methods which aim to alleviate anxiety can be tested by giving such questionnaires before and after an intervention. An investigator can then judge whether it has made a difference to patients' subjective feelings.

The cognitive side of anxiety

These questionnaires can provide a useful measure of a patient's anxiety level. However, another important way of gauging fear is to ask patients what they think about while in the chair or in the waiting room. It seems that highly anxious patients often dwell upon the worst possible outcomes they can imagine, thinking, for example, that the appointment is likely to result in intense pain, or that the dentist will discover that there is a vast amount of work needed. This kind of catastrophic thinking can be connected to a hypersensitivity to danger signs in the environment. An anxious patient may be very vigilant to any indication of threat such as the sight or sound of the drill, the wearing of a mask, or comments passed between members of the dental team. A simple question, such as 'What do you think might happen today?" could be very useful.

Physiological arousal

Another component of anxiety involves such autonomic signs as a higher pulse rate, dryness of the mouth and the release of stress hormones. Simpson et al. (1974) provide an illustration of how physiological variables are related to dental stress. Electrodes were placed on the forearms of children when they arrived for their first dental visit. After taking baseline measures before the dentist arrived, they monitored changes in heart rate and galvanic skin response to various procedures. The results for the children's heart rate are shown in Table 3.3. When the dentist changed into his white coat, for instance, the children's heart rate increased by 10 beats/min over baseline and it was 12 beats/min higher when the dental chair was raised. When the examination was finished, their hearts were beating an average of 3 beats/min below baseline. The results for skin conductance were similar.

The direction of the relationship between physiological arousal and subjective feelings of anxiety is far from clear. There is disagreement amongst psychologists as to whether arousal is a cause of feelings of

Table 3.3 Average changes in heart rate from baseline in the dental setting in children visiting for the first time

Activity	Change in heart rate (beats/min)
Dentist changes into a white coat	+10
Statement 'I am a dentist'	+15
Elevation of dental chair	+12
Adjustment of lamp	+10
Intra-oral examination	−1
End of examination	−3

From Simpson et al. (1974), with permission.

anxiety or a response to them. The problem is that few physiological signs are specific to particular emotions, in that the same signs might be shown for anger or exertion as for anxiety. Some psychologists argue that people first find that their hearts are racing and that they are perspiring and then interpret these signs according to the situation. In the dental chair they could be interpreted as anxiety while on the sports field as signs of exertion. Other psychologists contend that it is the other way around: that physiological arousal is a consequence of anxiety. A person may feel anxious about a situation and this then results in arousal, perhaps through adrenaline and catecholamine release.

Behaviour

A final component of anxiety is motor behaviour, which can take several forms. Behaviour problems shown by children (e.g. pushing the instruments away, refusing to open the mouth) are sometimes considered to be manifestations of anxiety. One method for assessing the amount of disruptive behaviour in children is a 4-point scale developed by Frankl et al. (1962). A child is placed in one of four categories according to the following criteria:

1. Definitely negative: Refusal of treatment, over-resistance and hostility, extreme fear, forceful crying, and massive withdrawal or isolation or both.
2. Slightly negative: Minor negativism or resistance and minimal to moderate reserved fear, nervousness or crying.
3. Slightly positive: Cautious acceptance of treatment, but with some reluctance, questions or delaying tactics, moderate willingness to comply with dentist.
4. Definitely positive: good rapport with operator, no sign of fear, interested in procedures and appropriate verbal contact.

It is preferable to be more precise than this. Melamed et al. (1975) listed a large number of behaviours which were considered to be fear-induced reactions to the dental surgery, as shown in Table 3.4. Instead of categorizing children on the basis of an overall impression, as Frankl et al. did, they clearly specified which reactions they would include and *time-sampled* their occurrence. Every 3 min the researcher indicated whether each of these had occurred. A child who was crying at any point during every 3-min interval would be given a higher score than someone who cried only once or twice. Each reaction was also weighted (as shown by the numbers in parentheses on the far left of Table 3.4), such that kicking the legs was scored as indicating twice as much anxiety as closing the eyes. In these ways an accurate description of the children's behaviour was gained.

Interobserver agreement
Whenever such rating scales are used it is important that there should be a high level of agreement between observers. Such agreement is certainly not to be taken for granted, since different people will use

Table 3.4 Some of the items used on a form for indicating the occurrence of fear-induced behaviour

	Successive 3-min observation periods
	1 2 3 4 5 6 7 8 9 10
Separation from mother	
(3) Cries	
(4) Clings to mother	
(4) Refuses to leave mother	
(5) Bodily carried in	
Office behaviour	
(1) Choking	
(2) Won't sit back	
(2) Attempts to dislodge instruments	
(2) Verbal complaints	
(2) Over-reaction to pain	
(2) White knuckles	
(2) Eyes closed	
(3) Cries at injection	
(3) Refuses to open mouth	
(3) Rigid posture	
(3) Crying	
(3) Dentist uses loud voice	
(4) Restraints used	
(4) Kicks	
(5) Dislodges instruments	
(5) Refuses to sit in chair	
(5) Leaves chair	

From Melamed et al. (1975), with permission.

different criteria and place different weightings on these. This problem is common whenever people's judgements are made. For example, Ludwick et al. (1964) were interested in comparing the quality of restorations undertaken by dentists and operating ancillaries in the US Navy. In order to do this, they asked experienced dentists to examine 152 restorations from the two groups, classifying them as excellent, good, fair or unsatisfactory. However, there was much disagreement between the seven dentists: in only 4% of the cases was there unanimous agreement, while in 9% the judgements ranged from excellent to poor. [Incidentally, the same might be said about assessments of dental students' work. In one study (Naitkin and Guild, 1967) there was much inconsistency between assessors when assigning grades. Sometimes the same grade was assigned for very different reasons.]

When rating behaviour, similar problems apply. If only one observer took ratings, he or she might use very different criteria for what constitutes 'rigid posture' or 'dentist uses a loud voice' than another observer. In order to reduce this problem, at least two observers should be used in psychological studies. Before the experiment proper is begun, they would make some observations and then compare notes. Through discussion they can specify where they disagree and ensure that they would use the same criteria during the experiment.

Avoidance of the dentist
To return to the discussion of the relationship between behaviour and anxiety, a person who is anxious about a situation can often cope simply by avoiding it. Many people would find parachuting anxiety-provoking, for example, yet this does not present a problem because there is no need to engage in such an activity. However, avoiding the dentist may be detrimental and there is some evidence that fear of dentistry affects appointment-keeping and attendance on a regular basis. Wardle (1982a) found a higher anxiety level in the patients who had not been to the dentist within the previous 2 years than those who attended within this time. It is possible to see how this could build up in a circular fashion: the longer a person delays visiting a dentist, the more likely it becomes that restorative work will be needed, thus raising the anxiety level (Kent, 1985).

A good way to assess the importance of anxiety on attendance would be to give a questionnaire to patients before they were due to attend and then see if they turn up. When Kleinknecht and Bernstein (1978) used this method they found support for the notion that anxiety affects attendance. Of those patients who had previously reported low fear, only 8% either cancelled or failed to show, while 24% of the high-fear patients missed their scheduled appointment.

Anxiety in the waiting room
Patients commonly report that their anxiety is at its height while they are waiting in reception rather than when they are actually in the chair. The anticipation of the event is often worse than the event itself. The reader may have experienced a similar feeling: anxiety about exams is often highest just before entering the examination hall. Once the exam begins anxiety subsides as attention is drawn towards answering the questions.

McTigue and Pinkham (1978) provide an interesting example of how dental anxiety can be shown in the waiting room. The children in this study (aged 3½–5½) were judged by their dentist as falling into one of three categories. Some showed definite negative behaviour in the surgery—crying, pushing the instruments away and so on. Others were definitely positive, being co-operative and interested in the dental work. Another group of children was more difficult to classify, sometimes being negative and sometimes positive, so that they seemed to fall between the other two groups. All children were later left to play in a room with a number of toys. Some of these toys were connected with dentistry, such as a miniature chair and plastic instruments. Others were non-dental, such as a tea set, a fire engine and a telephone. While they played the children were observed through a one-way mirror and the type of toy they chose and the amount of time they played with each were noted. The results showed that those children who showed negative behaviour in the dentist's chair chose the non-dental toys while those who showed the most positive behaviour played with the dental instruments. They would pretend to examine a doll's teeth, for example. Children in the intermediate group fell between the others in their choice of toys. All children could be assigned to their original groupings on the basis of their play, suggesting that this might be a potent means of distinguishing between anxious and non-anxious children before they enter the surgery.

Implications

These various components of anxiety are interdependent, but it is important to reiterate that there is no one-to-one relationship between them. One person who feels extremely anxious about dentistry may nevertheless attend regularly and be co-operative, while another person could be very disruptive. An illustration of this independence has been provided by a study in which heart rate recordings of children were taken while they were seated in the dental chair. Although accelerating heart rate was associated with active disruption by the children, other behavioural measures of anxiety showed little relationship with heart rate. For example, many of the children clenched their fists or forearms during examination but for them there was no corresponding increase in heart rate. For more than one-third of the children heart rate actually decreased during such behavioural displays of anxiety (Rosenberg and Katcher, 1976).

That these components of anxiety do not always correlate has several implications. One of these is theoretical, in that it is important in studying anxiety to take several measures sampling these different components. A practical implication for the dental practitioner is that he or she may find it difficult to judge patients' feelings from their behaviour. It may be remembered that when validating his DAS, Corah correlated patients' responses on the DAS with dentists' judgements of their anxiety. Although the correlations were statistically significant, indicating some validity, they were fairly low, about 0.42. This means that the dentists' judgements and the patients' self-reports were often dissimilar.

A second implication concerns the decision about how to help. Two patients may report that they feel anxious, but for one the main problem may seem to be behavioural (e.g. non-attendance), while for the other it may be physiological (e.g. a racing heart while in the waiting room). Perhaps the former patient would benefit from a different intervention than the latter, as discussed in the next chapter.

The causes of anxiety

One of the more obvious answers to the question of why people are anxious about dental treatment is that they anticipate some suffering. Wardle (1982a) asked her patients about the amount of pain they anticipated from several dental procedures (e.g. extraction, drilling, polishing). She also asked them about the amount of anxiety they felt about these procedures and then correlated the two scores together: all of the correlations were high (ranging from 0.65 to 0.85) with the exception of 'examination with a probe' ($r = 0.31$). Seventy-six per cent of the patients reporting high anxiety said that fear of pain was all or part of the reason for their fear. While 46% of the fearless patients expected their treatment to be painful, 70% of the fearful patients did so. These and other results suggest that a central reason for dental anxiety is anticipated pain.

However, this does not provide a full understanding of dental anxiety. First, it does not explain why many people who expect to experience pain do not report anxiety. Furthermore, this explanation assumes that anxiety is a result of pain, either expected or experienced, such that: pain leads to anxiety. Another possible explanation of this relationship is that anxiety leads to pain. Or perhaps the relationship is circular, so that anxiety leads to pain leads to anxiety, and so on.

There are some studies which support this possibility that heightened anxiety can affect pain tolerance and pain threshold. Kleinknecht and Bernstein's (1978) project makes the point. As described above, they posted anxiety questionnaires to patients before they arrived at the surgery. As well as taking measures of attendance, they also asked the patients to indicate how much pain they experienced during their appointment. When the high- and low-fear groups were compared, the high-fear patients reported more pain than the low-fear patients. This was not due to the types of treatment procedures the groups underwent, since these were similar. In some instances, at least, pain can be seen as a result or a symptom of anxiety rather than its cause.

In this section of the chapter, four main lines of research on the causes of anxiety are considered. One approach has to do with what has been called 'preparedness'. This may make people vulnerable to the effects of uncertainty and negative experiences. It seems that biological differences are also important.

Preparedness

A first approach to the aetiology of anxiety involves the possibility that people are innately predisposed to become anxious about the dental situation. Although this may seem far-fetched, there is some indirect evidence for this. Epidemiological studies of the sources of anxiety indicate that people are much more likely to be anxious about some situations than others. For example, the prevalence of phobias of spiders, cats and dogs is remarkably high. Many people are also frightened about enclosed spaces. Although these animals and situations do not pose a realistic threat to well-being, phobias about some dangerous situations are rare. For example, very few people are phobic about travelling at high speeds on the roads, which poses a realistic threat.

One way of making sense of these findings is to suggest that people are innately 'prepared' to be fearful about and avoid objects which, in our evolutionary past, did pose a threat. Perhaps small animals carried a threat of disease and enclosed spaces may have been associated with being trapped. Evolution could have favoured 'anxious genes' because anxiety could have raised the chances of survival. Since we are not prepared in the same way to be anxious about travelling at 70 mph, such phobias are rare (de Silva, 1988).

It is possible to see a link with dentistry. Lying on one's back with an adult placing sharp instruments in the mouth 'should' in some sense be frightening. Anxiety might be heightened particularly if the adult is a stranger (patients often find the prospect of joining a new practice distressing because they are concerned that the dentist will have a 'rough manner'), or if the patient is a child (where there is a large disparity of strength). This attractive idea goes some way towards explaining the widespread occurrence of dental anxiety. It would also make patients vulnerable to any effects of uncertainty and negative experiences.

Uncertainty

Anxiety is sometimes characterized as 'fear of the unknown' and there are indications from laboratory experiments in psychology that uncertainty, itself, is anxiety-provoking. Epstein and Roupenian (1970) persuaded people to volunteer for an experiment which involved undergoing a series of unpleasant electric shocks. Some were told that the probability of receiving a shock on any one trial was 1 in 20, while others were told that the chances were 19 in 20. On the basis of commonsense, one would expect that the second group would be more anxious than the first, since their probability of receiving a nasty shock was much higher. In fact, the opposite occurred: on measures of skin conductance and heart rate, the 1 in 20 group showed higher anxiety than the 19 in 20 group. It seemed that those in the high-probability group resigned themselves to the pain, while those in the low-probability group could neither resign themselves nor dismiss the thought that the shock would occur.

That this kind of process might be operating in anxious dental patients is suggested by Wardle (1982b), who reported that many of the patients she interviewed expected some kind of pain to occur. If they did not feel any discomfort on one visit they would leave with the feeling that they had somehow got away with it. 'Any time now he will get the nerve, and then it will really hurt' was a common thought reported by these patients when they underwent treatment. The probability of pain might be low, but it could happen at any time and therefore could not be dismissed. It is the *perceived* risk of pain which is important here, and not necessarily the actual experience which matters. Although non-anxious patients typically make accurate predictions of the amount of pain they are likely to experience during invasive procedures, anxious patients usually overestimate the likelihood of discomfort (Kent, 1984; Arntz et al., 1990).

Previous learning

A third approach to the aetiology of dental anxiety involves learning processes. The contention here is that anxious patients have had some kind of previous experience which has led them to expect that dental care involves pain. The typical procedure used to study this possibility has involved first dividing patients into high- and low-anxiety groups. This may be done by questionnaire, by interviewing people about their feelings, or by direct observation of behaviour. The next step is to attempt to find differences in the experiences of these two groups of patients. Shaw (1975), for example, selected 100 anxious and 100 non-anxious children on the basis of their dentists' judgements of anxiety. On questioning the mothers of these children, she found that the anxious children were more likely to have had an extraction on their first visit to the dentist, many of them finding the experience traumatic. Lautch (1971) interviewed phobic and non-phobic patients about their previous experiences. In his sample of 34 phobics, all reported at least one previous traumatic experience with a dentist, while only 10 of the 34 non-phobics could remember such an incident. Of the phobic patients who had returned to the dentist at least once after the experience (30 patients), all reported further traumas but only one of the non-phobics did so.

At first sight, these studies suggest that previous direct experience is an important cause of anxiety, but caution is required before making this conclusion. An important difficulty in both of these studies is that the investigators relied on the respondents' memories for information. It would have been preferable if dental records were consulted because this would provide verification of their reports.

Another difficulty is that in other studies of intensely fearful patients, not all have been able to remember traumatic incidents, suggesting that other kinds of experience are important for some people. Indeed, in the Shaw study, many of the children who were anxious about extractions and restorations had no history of a traumatic event. Furthermore, some children who have never been to the dentist are anxious on their first visit.

Anxiety and attendance patterns
In fact, there is no simple or clear relationship between previous experiences and anxiety. Brown et al. (1986) found that a decayed/missing/filled teeth (DMFT) index was *negatively* related to self-reports of anxiety; children with the greatest experience with invasive procedures had the lowest level of anxiety. A similar pattern was found by Murray et al. (1989) who performed a particularly interesting longitudinal study. They analysed the dental records for children over a 3-year period and found that frequency of attendance was an important factor. Children who attended irregularly and who received some invasive procedure during that time showed an increase in anxiety, while the anxiety level for those who attended regularly and had such a procedure did not change. But children who did *not* receive any invasive treatment, whether or not they attended regularly, were the most anxious overall. The suggestion from both these studies is that receiving invasive treatment in the context of regular attendance can act prophylactically.

The family's anxiety
For some people, the learning involved in dental anxiety may have been more indirect, depending on the experiences of other people. Shoben and Borland (1954) and Fogione and Clarke (1974) were able to uncover a pattern of family experiences not limited to anxious patients themselves. In the fearful group there was a more unfavourable attitude towards dentistry amongst the patients' relatives and more reports of traumas experienced by these relatives. This result was replicated by

Shaw (1975) who also found that mothers of anxious children were themselves more anxious and were more likely to comment on previous distressing experiences. It may be that the anxious patients' relatives served as models, displaying to them the kinds of consequence they could expect from a visit to the dentist.

The strongest evidence for the importance of this factor comes from a study by Johnson and Baldwin (1968). They first gave the mothers of their young patients an anxiety scale to complete. They then made observations of the children while they were in the dental chair, rating their behaviour as being generally positive or negative. The results are shown in Table 3.5. Those mothers whose anxiety was high were more likely to have children who reacted negatively. Most of the children in the study were visiting the dentist for the first time so their behaviour could not have been due to direct experience.

Table 3.5 The number of children showing positive or negative behaviour in the dentist's chair as related to their mothers' anxiety scores

	Children's behaviour rating	
	Positive	Negative
Mothers' anxiety score		
High	4	25
Low	25	6

From Johnson and Baldwin (1968), with permission.

A subsequent study (Koenigsberg and Johnson, 1972) showed that the relationship between mothers' anxiety and children's behaviour held for the first visit (which was for examination) but not for subsequent ones (for restorations). It seemed that actual experience became more significant for the children rather quickly. While some studies have replicated the relationship between mothers' anxiety and children's behaviour, there are also some failures to replicate (Bailey et al., 1973; Klorman et al., 1979), indicating that this particular association can be weak.

The dentist's role
Bernstein et al. (1979) examined the role of previous experience in a slightly different way. They first divided university students into high- and low-fear groups on the basis of their answers to a dental anxiety questionnaire. The students were then asked to write an essay describing their visits to the dentist as children. These essays were to include 'the features and events associated with those visits which determine present attitudes'. Forty-two per cent of the high-fear group mentioned pain during early appointments as a factor in their present reactions to dentistry, compared to 17.4% of the low-fear students. While these proportions discriminate between the groups to some extent, there was still the 58% of high-fear students who did not cite pain as a factor and a sizeable minority of low-fear students who did experience pain.

This overlap could be clarified by considering another variable—the personality of the dentist. Half of the high-fear group mentioned negative behaviour on the part of the dentist as a factor in their feelings about dentistry, most of these students not citing pain as a reason at all. The dentists were considered 'impersonal', 'uncaring', 'uninterested' or 'cold'. Thus it was about equally likely that an uncaring dentist would be seen by the students as the reason for their feelings as would be experience of pain. Furthermore, of the low-fear group who had experienced pain as children, many found the dentist 'careful', 'patient' and 'friendly'. The effects of the pain seemed to have been mitigated by a caring and concerned dentist. This study suggests that the dentist had an independent effect on the students' feelings (i.e. cold or uninterested behaviour was enough to make some students feel negatively about dentistry) and an interactive effect (i.e. caring and warmth could obviate the long-term effects of early painful experiences).

Classical conditioning
Another way in which dental anxiety could be learned is through a process termed 'classical conditioning'. The early development of classical conditioning theory was due to Pavlov, a Russian physiologist working at the beginning of the 20th century. In his original studies, he was interested in the digestive system, using dogs as his subjects. While giving food to his animals he noticed that after several feedings they would begin salivating even before they tasted the food. Sometimes their digestive systems would begin to work at the sight of the handler who fed them. The animals had learned, on the basis of past experience, that there was an association between the sight of the food and actually tasting it.

Pavlov began experimenting with this phenomenon, presenting lights or tones to the animals whenever they were fed. After several pairings of food and light, for example, the dogs would begin salivating to the light alone, in the absence of food. The light could then be paired with a tone and then this, too, would elicit salivation. He hypothesized that there could be many such associations between biologically significant events (e.g. food, water) and neutral stimuli in the environment and that this could account for much of human learning.

While psychologists today would consider this an oversimplification and would place more emphasis on other kinds of learning, there are several indications that classical conditioning is important in the learning of fears and anxiety. That it can be used to explain some fears has been demonstrated by Watson and Raynor (1920). In a much-quoted experiment, they showed a young child, called Albert, a white rat. At first Albert seemed very interested in the rat and wanted to play with it. Then, Watson and Raynor paired a loud aversive noise (a hammer striking a steel bar) with each presentation of the rat, so that every time Albert saw or touched it he would also hear the unpleasant noise. After only six pairings, Albert began to be distressed at the sight of the rat in the absence of the noise. The distress generalized to other white furry objects, such as a white rabbit, cotton wool and a fur coat. It seemed that Albert had learned to become afraid of the rat and other similar objects as a result of the pairing of a loud noise with the animal.

It may be that other fears, including fears about dentistry, sometimes develop in the same way. A person may have felt distressed when given an injection in the past, so that injections have become associated with pain. The experience may not even have occurred at the dentist's surgery: a patient might have been fearful when visiting a doctor (someone else who gives injections and who wears a white coat) and this fear could generalize to the dental setting. There was some supporting evidence for this kind of learning in Shaw's (1975) sample of dentally anxious children. In another report involving these same children (Semet, 1974), significantly more of the anxious children had a history of hospital admissions and negative attitudes towards the care they were given in hospital. It seemed as though their experiences with medical care generalized to dentistry. Gale and Ayer (1969) illustrate how fears can generalize in odd and surprising ways. They describe one patient who was very frightened of the dental chair who later became frightened of the chairs in hairdressers.

Thus, previous learning can take many forms. Experiences with pain may be important in developing anxiety about visits to the dentist, but the relationship between past experience and current anxiety is very complex. Other factors, such as attendance pattern and encounters with dentists who were seen as uncaring and unfriendly, can modify the meaning of a painful visit. In many cases the learning may have occurred more indirectly. A patient's friends and relatives provide models, giving expectations about how much discomfort a person might feel at the dentist's surgery. Fear can also generalize from one setting to others which appear similar in some way, so that a traumatic experience in a medical setting may generalize to dentistry.

Biological differences

Another approach to the aetiology of anxiety involves the possibility that some people are more predisposed to become anxious or to learn anxiety responses than others because of innate biological mechanisms. Biological differences could affect dental anxiety if some people had a lower pain threshold or lower pain tolerance than others. This could result in a greater likelihood of pain being experienced in the past and thus higher anxiety about experiencing it in the future. Another possibility relates to the classical conditioning approach. Pavlov's work was based on a biological viewpoint, stressing the importance of physiological responses to environmental stimuli. Since arousal is an important component of anxiety, it may be that individual differences in anxiety are due to differences in 'arousability'.

Neuroticism
Research on the relationship between physiological activity and personality characteristics has been conducted by Hans Eysenck. One of the characteristics he uses in describing people is called 'neuroticism', a term which has come to have many unfortunate connotations. People who answer in the affirmative to questions such as 'Are you moody?' and 'Do you often feel fed up?' would score high on the neuroticism

scale of Eysenck's (1967) questionnaire called the Eysenck Personality Inventory (EPI). Eysenck argues that personality is firmly based on innate, genetically determined mechanisms. People who score high on the neuroticism (N) scale are said to have autonomic systems which, once aroused, persist in a high state of arousal for long periods. This could result in a greater likelihood of classical conditioning occurring in high neuroticism scorers.

There is considerable evidence that scores on the N scale are linked to anxiety levels. A test of the importance of this factor is provided by a study which compared the N scores of regular attenders with those of patients who had avoided the dentist for long periods. The avoidant group consisted of patients who volunteered for a treatment programme designed to reduce dental anxiety. The comparison group was made up of patients who had identified themselves as regular attenders and whose dentists considered them to be fearless and co-operative.

When the EPI was administered to these two groups, those in the avoidant group gave significantly higher scores on the N scale than the regular attenders. An interesting finding was that part of the effect appeared to be due to the low-fear group giving lower N scores than the general population, so that the difference was not due wholly to the elevated scores of the avoidant group (Klepac et al., 1982). Because neuroticism seems to be linked with physiological characteristics, these results suggest that anxiety (or lack of it) can sometimes be explained by reference to innate mechanisms.

Childhood characteristics

Children vary in many ways. Some are more easily distracted from tasks than others; some are predominantly happy while others are more moody, and so on. While experiences are of course important in affecting such characteristics, there is now good evidence that they are partly genetically determined. They can emerge from a young age and persist over many years. Two important characteristics are known as 'approach-withdrawal' and 'adaptability'. A child who responds positively to a new situation (by smiling and moving towards it) can be contrasted with a child who responds negatively (by fussing and pulling away). Furthermore, some children adapt quickly to new situations while others take much longer.

Williams et al. (1985) showed the relevance of these characteristics to dentistry when they compared children who had been referred to a dental hospital because of a history of treatment refusal with those who were generally co-operative. The referred children were found to be more likely to withdraw from novel situations in general and to have difficulty in adapting to change. This suggests that such children will have more problems with entering the dental office even in the absence of any negative experience and will require a more gradual introduction.

Some conclusions

Generally speaking, it seems that a number of factors contribute to dental anxiety (Freeman, 1985). It may be that the dental situation is inherently anxiety-provoking, since it involves a patient lying in a vulnerable position. In addition, uncertainty may be significant for some people, while prior learning and innate factors may explain its presence for others. It is also possible that these factors have a cumulative effect: an individual who has a biological propensity to become anxious, who has relatives who are themselves anxious and communicate their worries, who attends irregularly and who has an early discomforting experience with dentistry may become much more likely to fear the dental setting than a person who has only one of these factors.

Summary

'Anxiety' is a term which has been used in a number of ways by different psychologists. Some have concentrated on the situational aspects of anxiety. Where dentistry is concerned, extraction, drilling and injection are the most anxiety-provoking features. There are important individual differences in how people react to these procedures, however, and several questionnaires have been developed to measure the amount of subjective anxiety a patient feels. The State–Trait Anxiety Inventory distinguishes between trait anxiety (a long-term discomfort) and state anxiety (which depends on the particular situation). There are several questionnaires designed specifically for dental patients, such as the Dental Anxiety Scale.

Anxiety can be manifested in several ways. Physiological arousal may occur, signalled by a high pulse rate or sweating. Behaviourally, children might show their anxiety by refusing to co-operate when in the dental chair while adults may be more likely to miss appointments or refuse to attend altogether. Scores on subjective, physiological and behavioural variables do not always agree, indicating that these components may operate independently of each other.

Patients often report that their anxiety stems from a fear of pain, but this does not provide a complete explanation since many people who expect pain do not seem anxious. Several theories have been put forward to explain the development of anxiety: some patients may be anxious because they are uncertain about what they will experience; others may have had a past experience with dentistry which has led to anxiety; others may be particularly vulnerable to learning anxiety responses. It could be useful to consider all of these influences when attempting to alleviate anxiety, the topic of the next chapter.

Practice implications

1 Different people show and experience anxiety in different ways, so it is not always possible to tell how anxious a patient might be. Anxiety levels might be higher in the waiting room, so that a receptionist's judgement could be useful.
2 Anxiety can 'run in families', so that a new child patient might experience a similar level of anxiety as a parent.

3 Because the dental setting may be inherently anxiety-provoking, the development of trust is crucial.
4 A gradual introduction might be especially helpful for children who have trouble entering or adapting to new situations.

References

Agras S., Sylvester D., Oliveau D. (1969) The epidemiology of common fears and phobias. *Compr. Psychiatry* **10**, 151–6.
Arntz A., van Eck M., Heijmans, M. (1990) Predictions of dental pain: the fear of any expected evil is worse than the evil itself. *Behav. Res. Ther.* **28**, 29–41.
Bailey P. M., Talbot A., Taylor P. P. (1973) A comparison of maternal anxiety levels with anxiety levels manifested in the child dental patient. *J. Dent. Child.* **40**, 25–32.
Bernstein D. A., Kleinknecht R. A., Alexander L. D. (1979) Antecedents of dental fear. *J. Public Health Dent.* **39**, 113–24.
Brown D.F., Wright F.A., McMurray N.E. (1986) Psychological and behavioural factors associated with dental anxiety in children. *J. Behav. Med.* **9**, 213–17.
Corah N. L. (1969) Development of a dental anxiety scale. *J. Dent. Res.* **48**, 596.
Corah N. L., Gale E. H., Illig S. (1978) Assessment of a dental anxiety scale. *J. Am. Dent. Assoc.* **97**, 816–19.
Curson I., Coplans M. P. (1970) The need for sedation in conservative dentistry. *Br. Dent. J.* **125**, 18–22.
Epstein S., Roupenian A. (1970) Heart rate and skin conductance during experimentally induced anxiety. The effect of uncertainty about receiving a noxious stimulus. *J. Pers. Soc. Psychol.* **16**, 20–8.
Eysenck H.J. (1967) *The Biological Basis of Personality*. Springfield, Illinois: Thomas.
Fogione A. L., Clarke R. E. (1974) Comments on an empirical study of the causes of dental fears. *J. Dent. Res.* **53**, 496.
Frankl S. N., Shiere F. R., Fogels H. R. (1962) Should the parent remain with the child in the dental operatory? *J. Dent. Child.* **29**, 150–63.
Freeman R. (1985) Dental anxiety: a multifactorial aetiology. *Br. Dent. J.* **159**, 406–8.
Gale E. N. (1972) Fears of the dental situation. *J. Dent. Res.* **51**, 964–6.
Gale E. N., Ayer W. A. (1969) Treatment of dental phobias. *J. Am. Dent. Assoc.* **73**, 1304–7.
Jackson E. (1978) Patients' perceptions of dentistry. In *Advances in Behavioural Research in Dentistry* (Weinstein P., ed.). Department of Community Dentistry: University of Washington.
Johnson R., Baldwin D. C. (1968) Relationship of maternal anxiety to the behaviour of young children undergoing dental extraction. *J. Dent. Res.* **47**, 801–5.
Kagan J., Havemann E. (1976) *Psychology. An Introduction*. New York: Harcourt, Brace, Jovanovich.
Kent G. (1984) Anxiety, pain and type of dental procedure. *Behav. Res. Ther.* **22**, 465–9.
Kent G. (1985) Cognitive processes in dental anxiety. *Br. J. Clin. Psychol.* **24**, 259–64.
Kleinknecht R. A., Bernstein D. A. (1978) The assessment of dental fear. *Behav. Ther.* **9**, 626–34.
Kleinknecht R. A., Klepac R. K., Alexander L. D. (1973) Origins and characteristics of fear of dentistry. *J. Am. Dent. Assoc.* **86**, 842–8.
Klepac R. K., Dowling J., Hauge G. (1982) Characteristics of clients seeking therapy for the reduction of dental avoidance: reactions to pain. *J. Behav. Ther. Exp. Psychiatry* **13**, 293–300.
Klorman R., Michael R., Hilpert P. L. et al. (1979) A further assessment of predictors of the child's behaviour in dental treatment. *J. Dent. Res.* **58**, 2338–43.
Koenigsberg S. R., Johnson R. (1972) Child behaviour during sequential dental visits. *J. Am. Dent. Assoc.* **85**, 128–32.

Lautch H. (1971) Dental phobia. *Br. J. Psychiatry* **119**, 151–8.
Lewis H. A. (1957) Unconscious castrative significance of tooth extraction. *J. Dent. Child.* **24**, 3–16.
Ludwick W. E., Schnoebelen E. O., Knoedler D. J. (1964) *Greater Utilization of Dental Technicians. II. Report of Clinical Tests*. Mimeograph. Dental Research Facility, US Naval Training Center, Great Lakes, Illinois.
McTigue D. J., Pinkham J. (1978) Association between children's dental behaviour and play behaviour. *J. Dent. Child.* **45**, 218–22.
Melamed B. G., Weinstein D., Hawes R. et al. (1975) Reduction of fear-related dental management using filmed modeling. *J. Am. Dent. Assoc.* **90**, 822–6.
Murray P, Liddell A and Donohue J. (1989) A longitudinal study of the contribution of dental experience to dental anxiety in children between 9 and 12 years of age. *J. Behav. Med.* **12**, 309–20.
Naitkin E., Guild R. E. (1967) Evaluation of pre-clinical performance. *J. Dent. Educ.* **31**, 152–61.
Rosenberg H. M., Katcher A. H. (1976) Heart rate and physical activity of children during dental treatment. *J. Dent. Res.* **55**, 648–51.
Segal H. (1986) Categories of emergency patient. *Gen. Dent.* **34**, 37–42.
Semet O. (1974) Emotional and medical factors in child dental anxiety. *J. Child Psychol. Psychiatry* **15**, 313–21.
Shaw O. (1975) Dental anxiety in children. *Br. Dent. J.* **139**, 134–9.
Shoben E. J., Borland L. (1954) An empirical study of the aetiology of dental fears. *J. Clin. Psychol.* **10**, 171–4.
de Silva P. (1988) Phobias and preparedness: replication and extension. *Behav. Res. Ther.* **26**, 97–8.
Simpson W. J., Ruzicka R. L., Thomas H. R. (1974) Physiologic responses to initial dental experience. *J. Dent. Child.* **41**, 465–70.
Speilberger C. D., Gorsuch R. L., Lushene R. E. (1983) *STAI Manual for the State-Trait Inventory*. Palo Alto: Consulting Psychologists Press.
Todd J. E., Walker A. (1980) *Adult Dental Health in England and Wales*. London: HMSO.
Todd J. E., Walker A., Dodd P. (1982) *Adult Dental Health, United Kingdom*. London: HMSO.
Tullman G. M., Tullman M. J., Rogers B. J. et al. (1979) Anxiety in dental patients: a study of three phases of state anxiety in three treatment groups. *Psychol. Rep.* **45**, 407–12.
Venham L. I. (1979) The effect of mother's presence on child's response to dental treatment. *J. Dent. Child.* **46**, 219–25.
Wardle J. (1982a) Fear of dentistry. *Br. J. Med. Psychol.* **55**, 119–26.
Wardle J. (1982b) Management of Dental Pain. Paper presented at the British Psychological Society Annual Conference, York, 1982.
Watson J. B., Raynor R. (1920) Conditioned emotional reactions. *J. Exp. Psychol.* **3**, 1–14.
Williams, J.M.G., Murray J., Lund C., Harkiss B., and de Franco A. (1985) Anxiety in the child dental clinic. *J. Child Psychol. Psychiatry* **26**, 305–10.

Chapter 4

Alleviating anxiety

The previous chapter considered research on two aspects of anxiety. The first was a discussion of the four components—the situation, subjective reports, physiological arousal and behaviour—which have proved useful in understanding the nature of anxiety. The second part of Chapter 3 considered the causes of anxiety. Patients' concerns are often focused on pain, but the dentist's personality, the uncertainty of dental care, previous learning experiences and biological predisposition can be important influences on these worries.

Preventing anxiety

Many clues about how to alleviate anxiety in dental patients can be gained from that research. Perhaps the best method is good prevention. Since negative experiences can sometimes lead to future anxiety, a reduction in the need for extractions and fillings would be a priority. Here the benefits of fluoridation of public water supplies and the importance of involving parents in their children's diet and oral hygiene habits become clear. If dental care is given on a regular basis and restricted to examination and cleaning, then early traumatic experiences can be eliminated to a large extent.

For children, the most important preventive measure is the provision of an environment in which they feel safe and trusting. This cannot be achieved immediately, nor does it rely simply on the dental staff doing the 'right thing'. It is important to take each individual child's needs into account by listening to and reacting to his or her communications. Many dentists argue that the actual accomplishment of treatment is always secondary to the establishment of trust when a new patient enters the office.

Although some people are frightened of injections, it is probable that the use of local anaesthetics has made a significant contribution to the reduction of dental anxiety amongst the public. Many older patients have reported that although they were very frightened of dentistry when younger, repeated visits over their lifetime have relieved their anxiety. This can be explained through extinction: patients who had been very anxious about dental care because it was associated with pain in the past may have come to learn that this association is no longer present after a series of pain-free visits.

78 The Psychology of Dental Care

Persistent anxiety

Where anxiety has developed and persists, however, several kinds of procedure might be followed. For those patients who feel pain despite local anaesthetics, psychological methods have been developed to lessen this discomfort, as discussed in the next chapter. Other patients who have found the behaviour and attitudes of their dentist worrying may be helped if the dentist can act in such a way as to relieve these apprehensions. One patient might be anxious because he or she is uncertain about what procedures a treatment may involve, while another might be concerned lest the dentist criticizes oral hygiene habits. Some studies on aspects of the dentist–patient relationship are discussed here, others in Chapter 7.

Pharmacological approaches
Pharmacological methods of anxiety relief provide another possibility. A general anaesthetic can be used in extreme cases but is generally considered to be inappropriate for most cases of anxiety. Many dentists are reluctant to use it partly because of the dangers involved and partly because it does not help the patient to come to terms with anxiety and learn how to cope with it.

An alternative pharmacological method is relative analgesia, which involves the inhalation of a mixture of nitrous oxide and oxygen. Roberts et al. (1979) studied the effects of relative analgesia on 65 children between 4 and 17 years of age, all of whom had shown unco-operative

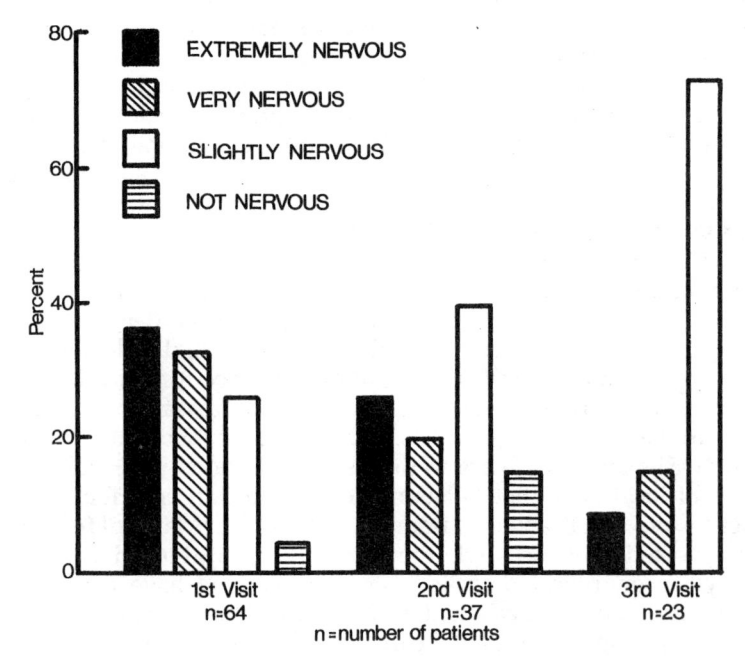

Figure 4.1 Assessment of anxiety at the beginning of each visit for children given relative analgesia. From Roberts et al. (1979), with permission.

behaviour in the dental chair. As the children arrived for their appointments their anxiety was judged as being uncontrollable, extremely nervous, very nervous, slightly nervous or not nervous. The amount of anxiety shown by the children as they arrived for their three visits is shown in Fig. 4.1. At the beginning of the first visit over 70% of the children were rated as being extremely or very nervous, but by the beginning of the third visit only 25% of the remaining children (some had completed treatment) were so judged. Co-operation improved in over 90% of the patients during this time and there was no indication of any adverse physiological effects. A follow-up of these children indicated that most were able to accept treatment at a later date without nitrous oxide sedation. Thus it would seem that this technique has some rehabilitative properties.

Hall and Edmondson (1983) have reported that intravenous diazepam, a tranquillizer, can have significant long-term effects on patients' fears. Of 70 phobic patients, 65 completed the initial course of treatment (for 2 treatment was abandoned and 3 were rendered edentulous). Of the 49 patients who could be traced 5 years later, only 3 had had no further dental care since the initial treatment. Thirty were receiving treatment with local anaesthesia only, while 16 still required intravenous sedation.

These pharmacological approaches can be helpful (Ryder and Wright, 1988, provide a useful review), but the purpose of this chapter is to discuss some psychological methods of alleviating anxiety. In the longer term they can be of greater benefit (Berggren and Linde, 1984). Just as psychologists have explored ideas about how dental anxiety is acquired, so, too, have they tested ways in which it might be lessened. These techniques are based on the research outlined in the previous chapter (which should be read before this one), indicating that uncertainty, previous learning and physiological arousal are involved in the aetiology of anxiety. By removing or reducing their influence, anxiety may be alleviated. This is, of course, an advantage to the dentist as well, in that the time invested in helping anxious patients may be rewarded by fewer disruptions to scheduling and more satisfying relationships. A variety of techniques are discussed below. One method which is becoming increasingly popular amongst dentists—hypnosis—is covered in the next chapter on pain, but it can be effective in reducing anxiety as well.

Some basic principles
Four central ideas underlie all of the treatments discussed in this chapter. They are as follows:

1 The methods provide the patient with increasing degrees of experience with the dental situation.
2 Exposure to the situation is increased gradually, so that the patient's coping strategies are not overwhelmed.
3 The aim is to help the patient manage his or her anxiety by increasing coping strategies or by changing perceptions of the dental setting.
4 Anxious patients are often ashamed of their difficulties and may be concerned about being judged negatively. Whatever the approach used, it is important to be accepting and non-evaluative.

80 The Psychology of Dental Care

Modelling

As discussed previously, modelling is based on the idea that people learn much about their environment from observing the consequences of others' behaviour. When we see someone rewarded for performing an action we will tend to repeat that action ourselves, while if someone is punished for it we will tend not to repeat it. In Chapter 2, modelling was shown to be a useful way of encouraging people to engage in preventive care at home. In the previous chapter it was suggested that modelling was one cause of anxiety. In our culture where dentistry is considered painful and something to be avoided, children in particular may come to fear a visit to the dentist because they have heard about negative experiences.

Conversely, modelling could be used to alleviate anxiety. If a patient could be shown that it is possible to visit the dentist, have treatment and then leave without undue distress, the anxiety might be reduced. Modelling could also be effective through the reduction of uncertainty. While observing a model undergo an examination or treatment, the patient would be gaining information about the kinds of equipment he or she will encounter and would learn which kinds of behaviour are acceptable.

Experiments on modelling

Melamed et al. (1975) tested the effect of modelling for children of 5–9 years of age, most of whom had little direct experience of dentistry. During the experiment, all were seen by the dentist three times: on the first

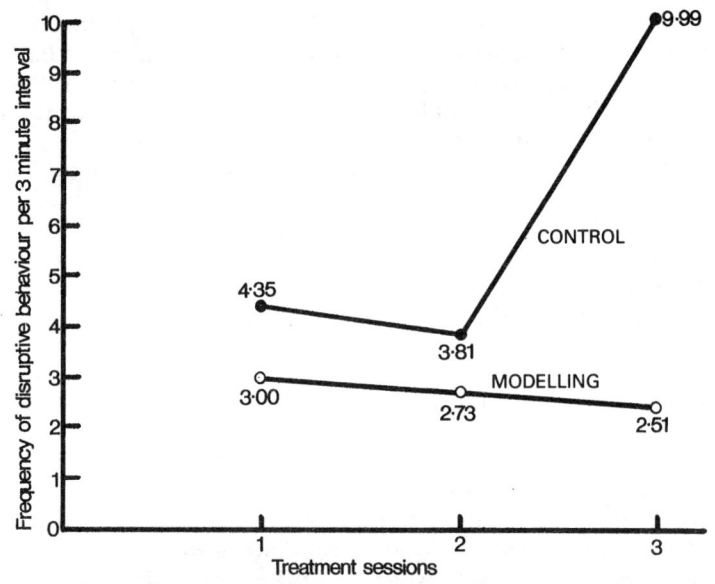

Figure 4.2 Frequency of disruptive behaviour in the modelled and control groups when (1) radiographs were taken, (2) the children's teeth were examined and (3) restorations were placed. From Melamed et al. (1975), with permission.

visit a radiograph was taken, an examination was given on the second and restorations were given on the third. Just before this last visit, one-half of the patients were shown a film of a 4-year-old child undergoing a restoration. The child on the film was praised by the dentist for his co-operative behaviour and was rewarded with a small toy at the end of the session. The remaining patients formed the control group, being asked to draw pictures for the same time interval as the film took to view.

Melamed et al. made several measures of anxiety during all three visits, including the amount and frequency of disruptive behaviour (e.g. crying, kicking, refusing to open the mouth). As shown in Fig. 4.2, the differences between the groups are insignificant at visits one and two, but a large difference was found on the third (treatment) visit. Those children who viewed the film continued to show a moderately low level of disruption despite the increased demands placed upon them. By contrast, the disruption shown by the control group children increased considerably.

Using films
Later research (e.g. Melamed et al., 1978) has indicated that care should be taken when developing and using such films. There is some evidence that for children with no prior experience of visiting the dentist, showing a film demonstrating procedures without a model could have a sensitizing effect, in that these children can become more disruptive. One important factor concerns the effects of including a model in the films as opposed to having the dentist simply describe what he or she was doing. Children who view films with a model report fewer fears and show less disruptive behaviour than children who view films demonstrating equipment, indicating that the presence of a model is important.

There are several other points. The model should show co-operation during treatment and be praised for this behaviour. The age of the model is significant, in that the best results are gained when the model is close in age to the target children. The model should also be shown leaving the surgery in much the same way as he or she arrived, thus indicating that the treatment does not have any lasting adverse effects. It is important that the dentist is portrayed as a caring individual who is concerned about the patient.

Using live models
It is not necessary to use films, however. Stokes and Kennedy (1980) describe how they arranged for some very disruptive children to arrive 10–15 minutes before their treatment was due to begin. The children were invited to observe a previous child being treated, who was praised and rewarded for being co-operative. Over four visits, the amount of disruptive behaviour shown by the children decreased by over two-thirds.

Family members can also be used if they have a low level of anxiety. In a case report, Klesges and Malott (1984) asked the mother of a 4-year-old dentally phobic girl to model coping behaviour, while Ghose et al. (1969) used siblings. In the latter study both siblings entered the surgery together and the younger child watched while the older was examined and treated. On the first visit the younger siblings were more likely to show positive behaviour when entering the surgery if the older sibling was present. On the second visit they were less disruptive during cavity preparation and amalgam preparation. Interestingly, these effects held only for children of 4 years of age—no differences were found for 3- and 5-year-olds—and were strongest when the sibling relationship was 'good' rather than 'fair' or 'poor'.

Participant modelling
Participant modelling requires more patient involvement. Here, they not only see a model undergo treatment but also go through the procedures themselves afterwards. In the first instance this can be simulated, the patient graduating to actual treatment later on. For example, Bernstein and Kleinknecht (1982) arranged for fearful patients to observe a model demonstrate the various steps needed in order to obtain professional care—telephoning a dentist, arriving at the surgery, receiving an oral examination and so on. Then the patients repeated each step themselves, only moving on to the next one when they felt comfortable. As each step was completed, they were praised for their progress. This approach seemed very useful, in that 87.5% of the patients, all of whom had avoided the dentist for up to 10 years, subsequently kept an appointment for treatment.

Reducing uncertainty

While modelling is an effective approach for reducing anxiety, it seems likely that at least some of the effect is due to the reduction of uncertainty and the reassurance given by a friendly and caring dentist. Since uncertainty raises anxiety, providing patients with information about their treatment would be expected to reduce it. Sometimes even small points of information, such as the expected length of the appointment, can be very helpful.

Many people will not understand the reason for dental procedures or the use of dental instruments. This is particularly true for children. For example, Eiser et al. (1983) found that more than half of the 6-year-olds they questioned did not know what an injection was. Children may also have misconceptions about dentistry: young children in particular may see the experience of discomfort as a punishment for past misbehaviour.

Tell Show Do

This is one method which has achieved much popularity as a way of introducing children to dental equipment and procedures. The *tell* phase involves an age-appropriate explanation of the procedures and the reasons for their use. The *show* phase is used to demonstrate a procedure, up to the point where the instrument is used. A cotton swab, rather than the needle, might be used to indicate the position of an anaesthetic injection. In a matter-of-fact way and with a minimum of delay the *do* phase is initiated. Throughout, the dentist seeks to relax the child and praise appropriate and co-operative behaviour. Unfortunately, in what seems to be the only experiment to have evaluated this approach (Howitt and Stricker, 1965) there was no evidence that it was effective for highly anxious children. Perhaps it would be more useful for children with lower anxiety.

Preparatory information

Other methods, which have involved preparing children and their parents for a first visit, have had some success. For example, Rosengarten (1961) posted preparatory information to some parents who were due to bring their children to the dentist for the first time. This included a short booklet to be read to the children. On their first visit no treatment or examination was given but instead the children were simply introduced to the office, the dentist and the hygienist. This preparation resulted in more co-operation being shown than for children not given the introduction, at least for those 3–4½ years of age.

It is not clear whether it was the visit or the booklet which was important for these children. In studies where parents have been given a preappointment letter alone (such as that shown in Table 4.1), the mothers have found them helpful (Wright et al., 1973) and there has been a reduced number of broken appointments (Hawley et al., 1974). However, there has been little effect on the actual behaviour of the children. In another study (Pinkham and Fields, 1976) where mother-and-child pairs were assigned to a control group, or given a reception room visit 1 week prior to the appointment, or given a visit and shown a videotape

Table 4.1 An example of a letter which could be sent to parents before their child's first dental visit

---

Your child's first dental visit

Dear

I am writing to you because I am pleased with the interest you are showing in your child's dental health by making an appointment for a dental examination. Children who have their first dental appointment when they are very young are likely to have a favourable outlook toward dental care throughout life.

At our first appointment we will examine your child's teeth and gums, and take any necessary X-rays. For most children this proves to be an interesting and even happy occasion.

All of the people on our staff enjoy children and know how to work with them. Parents play a most important role in getting children started with a good attitude toward dental care, and your co-operation is much appreciated. One of the useful things that you can do is to be completely natural and easy-going when you tell your child about the appointment with the dentist. This approach will enable him/her to view it primarily as an opportunity to meet some new people who are interested in him/her and want to help him/her to stay healthy.

Good general health depends in large part upon the development of good habits, such as sensible eating and sleeping routines, exercise, recreation and the like. Dental health also depends upon good habits, including toothbrushing, regular visits to the dentist and avoidance of excessive sweets. We will have a chance to discuss these points further during your child's appointment.

Best wishes, and I look forward to seeing you.

From Wright et al. (1973), with permission.

of procedures, the mothers' anxiety decreased as the number of interventions increased, but again no difference in the children's behaviour was found.

Preparation for extractions
When pre-visit preparation is given, it may be important to provide children with some time in order to accommodate themselves to dental procedures. In the first of two experiments, Baldwin and Barnes (1966) compared the reactions of children who had extractions with those whose treatment was more routine. In order to measure the stressfulness of these procedures, they used a 'draw-a-person' test (which is now rather outdated). The test involves asking the child to draw a figure of a person, including head, trunk, arms and legs. The size of the drawing was found to be related to the type of treatment. For those children undergoing a routine visit, the size of the drawings remained constant throughout: before treatment, just afterwards and at several follow-up visits. However, for those undergoing an extraction the size of the drawing was much smaller after they heard about the impending surgery than just before, and the drawings only gradually returned to their original size. This difference between the two groups was taken as an indication that the children given an extraction were in some distress.

Usually, children were told about the extraction 4–7 days before it was due to occur. Perhaps this was the cause of their distress: they had up to a week to worry about the extraction and time to become more and more concerned. Afterwards, this concern may have lingered on for a long time. Such a view would be consistent with the idea that children should not be told lest they worry about it. However, this idea does not tally with some observations that Baldwin and Barnes made on 2 children. Instead of the usual 4–7 days' notice, these children had their teeth removed within minutes of being told. In these cases, the drawings did not show the recovery in size until much later than usual, suggesting that they were experiencing continuing psychological difficulties. Perhaps the waiting period was, indeed, helpful.

In order to test the importance of this waiting period, Baldwin and Barnes arranged for a group of children to be given their extractions on the same day they were informed about them. They then compared their drawings with those by children given the usual week's warning. Instead of the typical recovery in size, the pictures of those informed just before the extraction remained constricted in size, beginning to increase only at the follow-up 1 month later. In other words, their recovery appeared to be much slower.

There was also some interesting interview data from the children and their parents. Every one of the children said that they would prefer to be warned in advance about dental extractions, expressed as a need to 'think about it', or 'get ready for it'. They said they wanted this time 'to get used to the idea' or 'to ask my friends about it'. Two of the children from the no-waiting group spontaneously remarked that they could never again be sure that when they went to the dentist he might not suddenly decide to take out a tooth.

By contrast, less than 50% of the parents thought their children should be told ahead of time. Some parents suggested that 'he'll just get scared' or 'why make her worry, there's enough time for that later in life'. Typical comments of those parents who felt that a waiting period was helpful were 'she's better off if she has time to think about it' and 'I always tell him what will happen'. Baldwin and Barnes suggested that one reason why children are pushed into surgery quickly is that the parents cannot cope with their own anxieties about it, as indicated by those who expressed such comments as 'I'm glad I'm not her today, I'm more nervous than she is'.

Amount of information

This idea of preparing patients for treatment by explaining what is going to happen to them well in advance is a most important one and will be discussed further in the next chapter on pain. It should be noted, however, that the children in the Baldwin and Barnes' study ranged from 8 to 14 years of age, so it is not certain that younger children would also benefit. It is also clear that it is possible to provide too much information for children on their first visit. It would be a mistake to work on the principle that if a little information is good, then more would be better. As mentioned earlier in connection with the study of Melamed et al. (1978), some of the children who had never visited the dentist before were more disruptive when they saw a film of a dentist demonstrating procedures and instruments without a model showing how to cope with them.

Swallow et al. (1975) found that the anxiety of inexperienced children was less when they were first interviewed in an adjoining room (with two easy chairs, no dental chair) and then treated in a room with the dental instruments hidden than when they were interviewed and treated in the standard surgery. Herbertt and Innes (1979) varied the amount of information about treatment procedures they gave to their patients. Some children received little treatment information, only being given a short lesson in dental health. Additional information was added for other groups until it was very detailed and thorough. The relationship between anxiety and information was curvilinear: too much or too little treatment information resulted in higher anxiety. When introducing a child to dentistry it seems important that a gradual approach should be used—one that allows a child to accomodate to the new environment slowly.

Personality

Another reason why it is important to be careful not to provide too much information about treatment concerns personality differences. From research in preparing patients for medical treatments, it seems that the recovery of some people is hindered by giving them more information than they want (Auerbach and Kilman, 1977). This information can over-ride patients' ways of coping with operations, making it more difficult for them.

The personality characteristic of locus of control is relevant here. It will be remembered from Chapter 2 that some people tend to believe that what happens to them is mainly a result of chance or fate and there is little they can do to change things. Such people are said to have an external locus of control. Other people, by contrast, tend to believe that events are largely under their own control and that they can affect outcomes, termed an internal locus of control. Auerbach et al. (1976) gave a questionnaire designed to measure locus of control to patients when they arrived at a dental clinic to have an extraction. They then showed two types of film. Some patients were shown a film containing general information: it described the clinic and some of the equipment they would encounter. Other patients were given much more specific information: they were told why extractions were sometimes necessary, a description of how the anaesthetic was given, the method of extraction was demonstrated and some ways to alleviate pain afterwards were suggested.

In order to measure anxiety, the oral surgeons rated how the patients reacted to the treatment. This judgement was based on how they responded to the anaesthetic, their degree of co-operation and the amount of pain they complained about. The scores of these various ratings were combined to give a total adjustment score and the results are shown in Fig. 4.3. The internal patients showed better adjustment during the extraction if they viewed the specific information film while this was not the case for the external patients. For them, there was a tendency to show poorer adjustment.

Thus, with both adults and children, it is important to be sensitive to the individual patient's requirements. It is important for the dentist to be open to the kind and amount of information which individual patients need. In many instances it is not what the dentist tells the patient which is important but rather what the dentist allows the patient to tell him or her which is crucial.

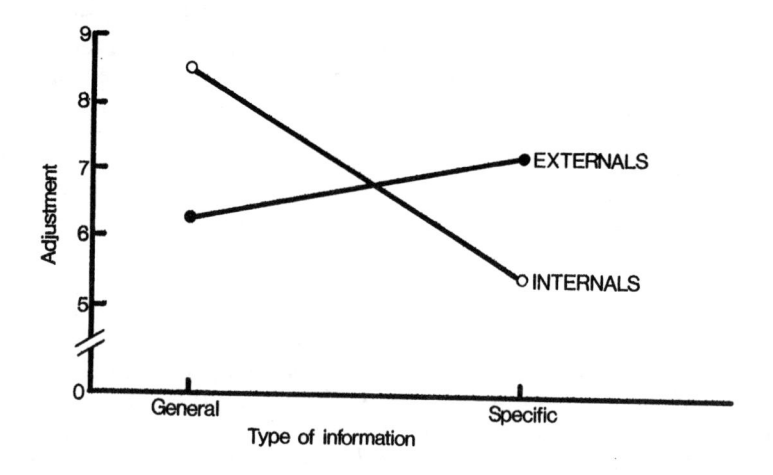

Figure 4.3 Adjustment shown by patients with external and internal locus of control when given either specific or general information about an extraction. A higher score represents poorer adjustment Adapted from Auerbach et al. (1976), with permission.

Enhancing control

One reason why uncertainty may be related to anxiety is that when people have little idea of what is going to happen to them they have little opportunity to alter their own or the dentist's behaviour. In other words, they have no control over the situation. Weinstein and Nathan (1988) argue that providing children with a sense of control is particularly important because of their feelings of vulnerability. They suggest that a sense of control can be enhanced by giving a multitude of small choices, such as asking children which side of the chair they would like to get up, whether they would like their top or bottom teeth cleaned first, offering a rest from procedures, and so on.

The idea that having control can reduce anxiety can be tested directly by giving patients a means of signalling their discomfort to the dentist. Corah (1973) explored this idea with children of 6–11 years of age. One group of children was given routine dental care. The other group was told that they could change their dentist's behaviour by pushing one of two buttons. When one button was pressed a green light would shine in front of the dentist. This could be used to indicate that the procedure was bothering patients but not so much that they wanted the dentist to stop working. Another button lit a red light and sounded a buzzer: this was to be used when the children wanted the dentist to stop for a short while until they felt more comfortable. On a galvanic skin response measure, the group of children given the buttons to push showed lower anxiety to highly stressful procedures (e.g. injection, drilling) but not to low-stress ones (e.g. placing amalgam).

However, this seems to be the only study in the literature where this approach has been shown to be useful in alleviating anxiety. In several others (Corah et al., 1978, 1979a; Thrash et al., 1982), providing patients with buttons which can be used to signal discomfort to the dentist had little effect. This is rather counterintuitive and is made even more puzzling by the results of many experiments relating control to pain. In that research area (discussed in the next chapter), telling patients that by pressing a buzzer or raising an arm they can signal the dentist to stop working has consistently reduced reported pain.

Emotional support

While the anxiety associated with uncertainty can be reduced by providing information, the dentist is also providing emotional support when he or she takes the time to explain the nature of procedures and treatment. There is the implicit message that the dentist is aware of the anxieties inherent in the situation and is attempting to reduce them. This provides some security and trust.

A study on children who were about to have a minor operation (Fassler, 1980) illustrates this more clearly. One group were given extensive preparation for their hospitalization. They were read a story about a child going to the hospital and given a set of hospital toys to play with which could be used to depict hospital scenes. The children were also encouraged to express any fears and doubts about their operation and any misconceptions were corrected. This intervention thus involved both factual information and emotional reassurance—how important was the emotional support? In order to look at this, another intervention was included in the study. A second group of children was given emotional support but no direct information. They, too, heard a story, were given toys to play with and engaged in conversation, but the conversation centred around school and friends rather than hospitalization, and the toys and story did not concern hospitals. The third group of children were given no additional emotional support or preparatory information.

All the children were then asked about their present feelings. The results for the three conditions are shown in Fig. 4.4: those given emotional support plus information reported the lowest anxiety, followed by those given emotional support alone, while the no-intervention group showed the highest anxiety level. Thus, emotional support alone had a beneficial effect on anxiety and this was further enhanced by giving preparatory information.

While few dentists will be able to spend so much time with their child patients, it is useful to recall the results of a study mentioned in the previous chapter. There, university students were asked to write an essay describing their visits to the dentist as children, including those events which influenced their present attitudes. The personality of the dentist was significant for the students, with many of them recalling their dentist as being either 'cold' and 'uncaring' or 'warm' and 'friendly'. Even in these relatively brief encounters the emotional support given by their dentists had a lasting effect on their feelings.

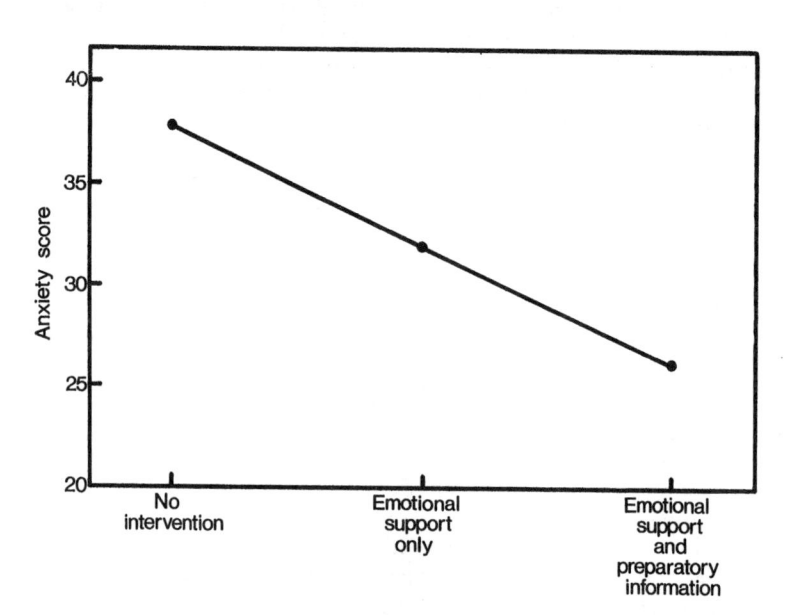

Figure 4.4 Anxiety scores for hospitalized children who had received no intervention, received emotional support, or received both emotional support and preparatory information. From Fassler (1980), with permission.

Parents in the surgery

It could be argued that the child's family is in the best position to offer emotional support and this raises the important question of whether a child's parents or siblings should be allowed in the surgery during treatment. There is now strong evidence that a parent should be encouraged to room-in with a child during hospitalization but there is no conclusive evidence concerning the effects of a parent's presence in the dental surgery. The argument against letting a parent attend is that the child is more likely to 'play up'. However, there is no evidence that disruption is more likely when a parent is present in the surgery. In some respects this might be considered an ethical rather than simply an empirical problem—does the dentist have the right to bar a parent who wishes to join the child in the surgery?

It may be that the absence of any effect in the studies in this area is due to the standard experimental procedure of randomly assigning parents and children to either present or absent conditions. As Venham (1979) puts it:

> Some children clearly received strong support and security from the mother's presence. On several occasions, a child grasped the mother's hand. On the other hand, several mothers clearly exhibited behaviour that would tend to increase the child's anxiety. They openly expressed fear of the dentist and specific dental procedures in front of their children and asked to avoid seeing the procedure. These mothers moved nervously in their chairs, hid their eyes, displayed exaggerated facial signs of fear and emitted sounds associated with fear and anxiety, all in full view of their children (p. 221.)

A more sophisticated experimental procedure, where the anxiety of the parent is taken into account, may indicate that a parent's presence is helpful when he or she is calm, but unhelpful if anxious. In the latter case the parent may require assistance, perhaps through some of the techniques discussed in this chapter. (Incidentally, several dentists have noted that anxious parents sometimes send their children to a dentist first in order to gauge the dentist's abilities. By doing everything possible to relieve any anxiety the child might feel, the parents' fears might also be reduced, making it possible for them to seek treatment for themselves.)

Relaxation

The idea behind the use of this kind of therapy is that anxiety is associated with certain kinds of physiological arousal—high heart rate, muscular tension and sweating. If a patient could be taught to control these signs of arousal, an important component of anxiety could be reduced.

Relaxation training

There are several methods for teaching relaxation, but the general aim is to induce muscle relaxation. One approach uses biofeedback (e.g. Miller et al., 1978), but the problem with this is that it requires specialist equipment and is probably no more effective than alternative methods.

The best known and validated method is called progressive muscle relaxation. The patient is asked to sit in a comfortable reclining chair. The therapist then asks the patient first to tense and then relax the major muscle groups in the body. The procedure often starts with the toes and then progressively works through the ankles, calves, thighs and so on. Slow and controlled breathing with the eyes shut is finally achieved. The exercise takes 15–25 min to complete and the patient would be asked to remain in this state for a further 10 min or so. For most people, this results in a general feeling of calm and relaxation, a feeling very different from that engendered by anxiety. After several training sessions people can generally relax themselves fairly quickly without the presence of the therapist.

This technique has been used in a wide variety of circumstances, perhaps most notably in preparation for childbirth. Lamb and Strand (1980) describe how they used it for dental patients who were scheduled for routine treatments. As they arrived, they were given the State–Trait Anxiety Inventory anxiety questionnaire, discussed in the previous chapter. One-half of the patients were then escorted to another room, seated in a reclining chair and asked to follow the instructions on an audiotape which explained the muscle relaxation method. After this 14-min tape, the patients were again asked to fill out the anxiety questionnaire

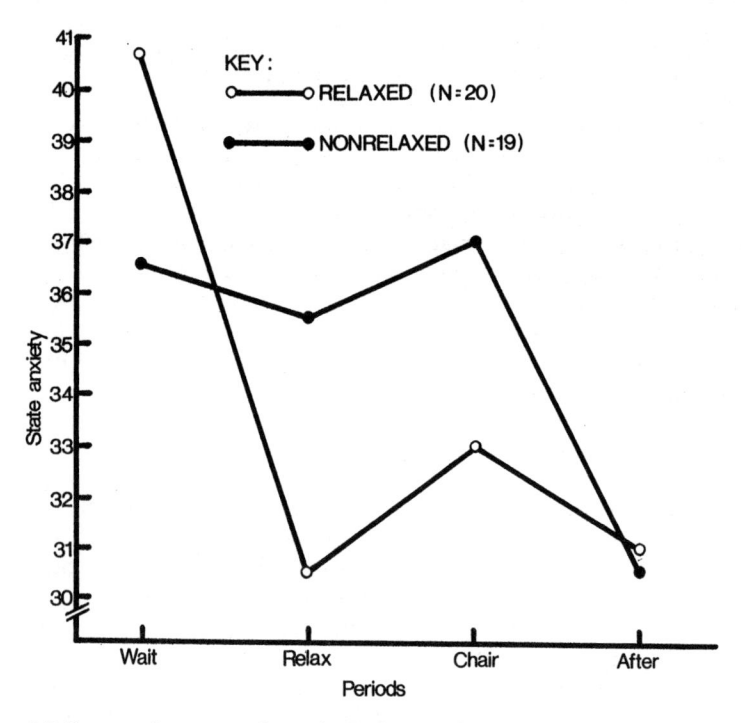

Figure 4.5 State anxiety scores for patients given and not given relaxation training. The anxiety of patients who heard a relaxation tape decreased before the treatment but the anxiety of the non-relaxed patients decreased only after treatment was completed. Adapted from Lamb and Strand (1980), with permission.

and then accompanied to the dental chair. When the dental treatment was completed, the anxiety questionnaire was filled out twice more, once according to 'how you felt while you were in the dentist's chair' and finally according to 'how you feel right now'. The other half of the patients were not given the relaxation exercise but were asked to fill out the questionnaires during the same time periods.

The results for the state anxiety measures are shown in Fig. 4.5. For the relaxation group, the scores dropped after hearing the tape and did not rise significantly during the dental treatment. By contrast, the group not given relaxation training showed no decrease in anxiety until they had left the chair. One problem with this study is that the control group received no special attention comparable to that given to the relaxation group. It may be that the anxiety scores for the relaxation group decreased not because of the training itself but rather because they received more care and attention. That is, the result may have been due to a placebo effect. It would have been preferable if the control group had received a similar amount of attention. Nevertheless, this study at the least shows that anxiety can be reduced with a minimum of intervention by clinicians with only a small amount of formal training. Nor did the intervention disrupt the patients' visit or the dentist's scheduling.

Systematic desensitization

The notion that patients could become less anxious about dentistry through repeated contacts is a familiar one: if an anxious patient finds that on several occasions nothing distressing occurs, the anxiety will eventually be reduced. However, this is rather haphazard. Nor does it apply to patients who are so frightened of dentistry that they refuse even to enter the surgery. In systematic desensitization (SD) the process is formalized and it can be used for severely anxious patients.

The technique may be best described by outlining a case study (Gale and Ayer, 1969). The patient was a 32-year-old male who had a history of avoiding the dentist. He was taken to a dentist at age 5 or 6, but tried to flee from the office. At 8 years of age, he refused to have any dental work done. At 18 he had one filling and then refused to return. Later, after a toothache lasting 3 weeks, he finally went to a dentist who placed him under general anaesthetic. Several teeth were removed and several restorations completed. Over the next 12 years or so he suffered repeated toothaches but had not seen a dentist. During SD, the patient was seen by a therapist for 9 sessions of about 1 hour each. At the first session the history was taken and relaxation therapy begun. In the second session further relaxation training was given and the patient was asked to list his fears about the restoration of his teeth. These fears were ordered in a hierarchy, as shown in Table 4.2. The least anxiety-provoking situation was thinking about going to the dentist while the worst was receiving two injections, one on each side. Another list was made for extractions. In the third session relaxation therapy was completed.

The next 6 sessions were devoted to pairing the relaxation with the items in the hierarchy. In SD this is done by asking the patient to relax as fully as possible. He is then requested to visualize the situations

Table 4.2 Hierarchy of patient's fears from least (1) to most (13) feared situation

1 Thinking about going to the dentist
2 Getting in your car to go to the dentist
3 Calling for an appointment with the dentist
4 Sitting in the waiting room of the dentist's office
5 Having the nurse tell you it's your turn
6 Getting in the dentist's chair
7 Seeing the dentist lay out the instruments, one of which is a probe
8 Having a probe held in front of you while you look at it
9 Having a probe placed on the side of a tooth
10 Having a probe placed in a cavity
11 Getting an injection in your gums on one side
12 Having your teeth drilled and worrying that the anaesthetic will wear off
13 Getting two injections, one on each side

From Gayle and Ayer (1969), with permission.

which he finds frightening, starting with the least frightening one. Whenever he feels anxious, the therapist instructs him to stop thinking about this situation and concentrate again on the relaxation. By pairing relaxation with the image, the situation begins to lose its anxiety-provoking properties. When the patient can visualize the least frightening situation without feeling anxious, he moves on to the next step of the hierarchy. This is repeated until he or she can think of the most frightening situation without becoming anxious.

SD was very successful with this particular patient. Just before the ninth session he made and kept an appointment with a dentist. Afterwards, all necessary dental treatment was completed and he found it 'relaxing'.

Cognitive approaches

While modelling is based on the idea that people can learn about the consequences of dental care from watching others and the various types of relaxation training serve to inhibit physiological arousal, cognitive strategies operate on a different principle. It seems that anxious dental patients often think about the worst possible consequences of dental care, of a 'Any time now he will get the nerve and then it will really hurt' kind. For many anxious patients, it is not a question *if* they will experience pain, but *when*. Once these anxiety-laden thoughts come to mind they seem to heighten a patient's anxiety level, so that a vicious circle develops. If these kinds of anxiety-provoking thoughts can be prevented, then the anxiety itself could be reduced. The studies discussed under 'Reducing uncertainty' earlier in the chapter could be included here since they also involve changing the way patients perceive the dental situation. In this section, two methods are outlined—distraction and cognitive modification.

Distraction

In this approach, the aim is to shift the patient's attention away from the dental setting and towards some other kind of situation. If patients are thinking about something other than the dental work, they are less likely to dwell on anxiety. It follows that the more a distractor captures the attention, the more effective it will be.

In one experiment (Corah et al., 1979a) adult patients who required at least two visits for restorations were studied. One group of patients was given no intervention: their dental treatment proceeded as usual. A second group was asked to listen to a relaxation tape during treatment, through headphones. The tape asked the patients to relax their muscles as in progressive relaxation, except that the jaw muscles were excluded because this would interfere with the dentist's work. A third group of patients were assigned to a 'perceived control' group. They were told that they could ask the dentist to stop the work by pressing a button which would sound a buzzer. The dentist would then pause until the patient was more comfortable. The patients in the remaining group were given a way of distracting their attention from the treatment. A ping-pong video game which they could play throughout the restoration was mounted on the ceiling above their heads. This served to shift their attention away from the dentist's work.

The relaxation and distraction conditions were equally effective in reducing discomfort for anxious patients and these two interventions were superior to the no-intervention condition. The 'perceived control' condition had a small and non-significant effect. In the second study (Corah et al., 1979b) many of the same results were found but there were some important sex differences. Distraction was generally more effective in reducing anxiety for men while relaxation was better for women.

Distraction for children
There is some disagreement as to whether distraction is an effective approach with children, with some studies finding that it is not helpful. However two reports indicate that the type of distractor and the way it is presented are crucial. Ingersoll et al. (1984a) encouraged children to view videotaped cartoons during treatment, but some children were told that the video would be switched off if they became unco-operative while for other children the video played regardless of their behaviour. The second condition had very little effect: their behaviour was similar to a control group who underwent treatment with no distractor available. However the amount of disruptive behaviour was halved in the group who were told that the availability of the cartoons was contingent on their behaviour. In a later study (Ingersoll et al., 1984b), audiotaped stories were used: this was even more effective than the cartoons, perhaps because the children tended to close their eyes in order to concentrate on the stories so that the sights as well as the sounds of treatment were excluded. These studies indicate that a distractor may be effective in changing behaviour only if there is some incentive, and some distractors are more effective than others.

Cognitive modification

While distraction aims to shift the patient's attention away from the distressing situation, the cognitive modification view is a very different one. Here the aim is to focus attention on the positive aspects of treatment. Instead of dwelling on possible negative consequences (e.g. 'Any time now he will hit the nerve'), the patient is asked to concentrate on some positive possibilities, such as 'The dentist has never hurt me before and she won't do it now' or 'Once this appointment is finished, my teeth will be clean and healthy'.

Nelson (1981) illustrated this method in a case study of a young girl with a dental phobia. He concentrated on the rehearsal aspect by first modelling coping self-statements (e.g. 'The dentist is really your friend') and then asked the girl to verbalize the statements herself. Several role plays were used in which they practised these statements. Over several appointments, anxiety decreased so that the girl was able to enter the dental setting with less anxiety and less disruptive behaviour.

Choosing between interventions

The evidence described thus far indicates that modelling, reducing uncertainty, providing emotional support, relaxation and the cognitive approaches are all effective in reducing anxiety. Most of these techniques have been tested on both normally and intensely anxious groups of patients. With such a variety of effective methods available, an important question concerns when to use one technique in preference to another. If one kind of intervention could be shown to be superior to other kinds, then perhaps this would be the treatment of choice for most patients.

There are several studies in which some patients have received one type of intervention (e.g. practice in the use of distraction) or another (e.g. preparatory information). In general, about 60–80% of patients are helped regardless of the therapy type and in most studies patients given some form of assistance are able to cope better than those given none.

Common factors in therapies

Some psychologists have argued that this similarity of treatment effectiveness is because most therapies have several features in common. The patient is given hope that his or her anxiety will be relieved, and the therapist is giving the patient time and attention which provide emotional support. These factors alone might be sufficient to reduce discomfort (Murray and Jacobson, 1971). Certainly, when the therapist is cold or business-like the effectiveness of these interventions is much reduced. Another argument is that patients who avoided the dentist in the past may want to test the effectiveness of their therapy by making and keeping a dental appointment. As one patient put it after completing therapy, 'I am very curious about how I will react when I go to the dentist' (Bernstein and Kleinknecht, 1982). Once they have made a visit they may find that the experience is not as distressing as they anticipated [e.g. 'I finally tried Novocain and when I realized that it didn't hurt to get a shot and that I couldn't feel anything while he was drilling, I felt stupid for being so afraid of getting my teeth filled' (Bernstein and Kleinknecht, 1982)].

Matching therapy to patient

Other psychologists contend that this similarity in effectiveness is due to the way in which these experiments have been designed. Patients are usually assigned to various therapies on a random basis, so that individual differences in age, personality or previous experiences are equally distributed across conditions. While such a procedure has advantages, it may be that certain types of therapy are more effective with certain types of people (Kiesler, 1971). Perhaps a patient whose anxiety is primarily behavioural in nature would receive most benefit from a participant modelling approach, while for another patient whose difficulty is more biologically based, a relaxation method would be better.

Patients' advice

Patients' own views are relevant. Many who are extremely nervous will expect or prefer some kind of pharmacological sedation (Lindsay et al., 1987), so that a dentist who prefers a psychological approach will need to take this into consideration. When O'Shea et al. (1986) asked patients what they would do if they were dentists to relieve anxiety, several methods were suggested, as shown in Table 4.3. There is a wide range of possibilities: asking individual patients about their preference may help in making an appropriate choice.

Table 4.3 Patients' advice on how to reduce anxiety

Provide an initial explanation of planned procedures
Provide an explanation and description of procedures as they are being performed
Instruct the patient to be calm
Warn that discomfort may occur at particular points in a procedure
Support the patient by showing concern and being reassuring
Help the patient redefine the experience away from pain by providing a new way of viewing the situation
Give the patient some control over procedures
Help the patient to cope, e.g. through breathing exercises
Provide a way of distracting the patient
Build trust
Show personal warmth
Start with minor things first

Clinical psychology

When a patient does not respond to such simple interventions as relaxation training or a gradual introduction to the dental office (or if the anxiety seems too intense even to attempt any intervention), referral to a specialist may be appropriate. Clinical psychologists have extensive training in the methods outlined in this chapter and can be contacted through the patient's general medical practitioner or privately. Subsequently the psychologist may ask for your co-operation in introducing the patient to the equipment or surgery.

Summary

Persistent anxiety in dental patients can be relieved in many ways. Modelling provides the patient with an opportunity to see others showing little distress while being treated and may be effective partly because it removes some of the uncertainty involved in dental care. Direct reduction of uncertainty is also effective: providing patients with clear information about the kinds of equipment and procedures they will encounter alleviates anxiety, particularly for those with an internal locus of control. It is important to remember, however, that it is possible to provide too much information for some patients, particularly children who may have difficulties in coping with the equipment found in the surgery. Emotional support is very important for this group of patients. Relaxation and systematic desensitization operate by reducing the physiological arousal associated with anxiety. Distraction can be another effective technique: by shifting the patient's attention away from the dentist's work, patients are less likely to think about the possibility of pain.

Practice implications

1 In order to prevent the development of anxiety, more attention should be given to the enhancement of trust than the completion of treatment for a new patient.
2 Siblings, parents and other patients can be used as models.
3 Although giving information can be helpful, avoid providing more detail than is needed.
4 Many patients use distraction. They can be helped in this if provided with attention-capturing materials such as audiotaped stories.
5 Patients have their own strategies for coping. These can be discovered and strengthened.
6 Consult a clinical psychologist if necessary.

Suggested reading

A further overview of this area is given in Rubin J.G. and Kaplan A. *Dental Phobia and Anxiety. The Dental Clinics of North America, Vol. 32.* (London, Saunders, 1988).

References

Auerbach S. M., Kendall P. C., Cuttler H. F. et al. (1976) Anxiety, locus of control, type of preparatory information and adjustment to dental surgery. *J. Consult. Clin. Psychol.* **44,** 809–18.
Auerbach S. M., Kilman P. R. (1977) Crisis intervention: a review of outcome research. *Psychol. Bull.* **84,** 1189–217.
Baldwin D. C., Barnes M. L. (1966) The psychological value of a pre-surgical waiting period in the preparation of children for dental extraction. *Trans. Eur. Orthodont. Soc.,* pp. 297–308.
Berggren U., Linde A. (1984) Dental fear and avoidance: comparison of two modes of treatment. *J. Dent. Res.* **63,** 1223–7.

Bernstein D. A., Kleinknecht R. A. (1982) Multiple approaches to the reduction of dental fear. *J. Behav. Ther. Exp. Psychiatry* **13**, 287–92.

Corah N. L. (1973) Effect of perceived control on stress reduction in pedodontic patients. *J. Dent. Res.* **52**, 1261–4.

Corah N. L., Bissell G. D., Illig S. J. (1978) Effect of perceived control on stress reduction in adult dental patients. *J. Dent. Res.* **57**, 74–6.

Corah N. L., Gale E. H., Illig S. J. (1979a) Psychological stress during dental procedures. *J. Dent. Res.* **58**, 1347–51.

Corah N. L., Gale, E. H., Illig S. J. (1979b) The use of relaxation and distraction to reduce psychological stress during dental procedures. *J. Am. Dent. Assoc.* **98**, 390–4.

Eiser C., Patterson D., and Eiser J.R. (1983) Children's knowledge of health and illness: implications for health education. *Child Care, Health Dev.* **9**, 285–92.

Fassler D. (1980) Reducing preoperative anxiety in children. *Patient Counsel. Health Educ.* **2**, 1304.

Gale E. H., Ayer W. A. (1969) Treatment of dental phobias. *J. Am. Dent. Assoc.* **8**, 130–4.

Ghose L., Giddon D., Shiere F. et al. (1969) Evaluation of sibling support. *J. Dent. Child.* **36**, 35–49.

Hall H., Edmondson H. D. (1983) The aetiology and psychology of dental fear. *Br. Dent. J.* **154**, 247–52.

Hawley B. P., McCorkle A. D., Witteman J. K. et al. (1974) The first dental visit for children from low socio-economic families. *J. Dent. Child.* **41**, 376–81.

Herbertt R. M., Innes J. M. (1979) Familiarisation and preparatory information in the reduction of anxiety in child dental patients. *J. Dent. Child.* **46**, 319–23.

Howitt J. W., Stricker G. (1965) Child patient responses to various dental procedures. *J. Am. Dent. Assoc.* **70**, 71–4.

Ingersoll B.D., Nash D., Blount R., Gamber C. (1984a) Distraction and contingent reinforcement with pediatric dental patients. *J. Dent. Child.* **51**, 203-7.

Ingersoll B.D., Nash, D., Gamber C. (1984b) The use of contingent audiotaped material with pediatric dental patients. *J. Am. Dent. Assoc.* **109**, 717–19.

Kiesler D. J. (1971) Experimental design in psychotherapy research. In *Handbook of Psychotherapy and Behaviour Change* (Bergin A. E., Garfield S. L., eds). London: Wiley.

Klesges R., Malott J. (1984) The effects of graded exposure and parental modeling on the dental phobias of a four-year-old girl and her mother. *J. Behav. Ther. Exp. Psychiatry* **15**, 161–4.

Lamb D. H., Strand K. H. (1980) The effect of a brief relaxation treatment for dental anxiety on measures of state and trait anxiety. *J. Clin. Psychol.* **36**, 270–4.

Lindsay S.J.E., Humphris G., Barnby G. (1987) Expectations and preferences for routine dentistry in anxious adult patients. *Br. Dent. J.* **163**, 120–4.

Melamed B. G., Weinstein D., Hawes R. et al. (1975) Reduction of fear-related dental management problems with use of filmed modelling. *J. Am. Dent. Assoc.* **90**, 822–6.

Melamed B. G., Yurcheson R., Fleece E. L. et al. (1978) Effects of film modelling on the reduction of anxiety related behaviour in individuals varying in level of previous experience in the stress situation. *J. Consult. Clin. Psychol.* **46**, 1357–67.

Miller M. P., Murphy P. J., Miller T. P. (1978) Comparison of electromyographic feedback and progressive relaxation training in treating circumscribed anxiety stress reactions. *J. Consult. Clin. Psychol.* **46**, 1291–8.

Murray E., Jacobson L. (1971) The nature of learning in traditional psychotherapy. In *Handbook of Psychotherapy and Behaviour Change* (Bergin A. E., Garfield S. L., eds). London: Wiley.

Nelson W.M. (1981) A cognitive-behavioural treatment of disproportionate dental anxiety and pain: a case study. *J. Clin. Child Psychol.* **15**, 79–82

O'Shea R.M., Corah, N.L., Thines T. (1986) Dental patients' advice on how to reduce anxiety. *Gen. Dent.* **11**, 44–7.

Pinkham J. R., Fields H. W. (1976) The effects of pre-appointment procedures on maternal manifest anxiety. *J. Dent. Child.* **43**, 180–3.

Roberts G. J., Gibson A., Porter J. et al. (1979) Relative analgesia: an evaluation of the efficacy and safety. *Br. Dent. J.* **146,** 177–82.

Rosengarten M. (1961) The behaviour of the pre-school child at the initial dental visit. *J. Dent. Res.* **40,** 673.

Ryder W., Wright P. (1988) Dental sedation. A review. *Br. Dent. J.* **165,** 207–16.

Stokes T. F., Kennedy S. H. (1980) Reducing child unco-operative behaviour during dental treatment through modelling and reinforcement. *J. Appl. Behav. Anal.* **13,** 41–9.

Swallow J., Jones J., Morgan M. (1975) The effect of environment on a child's reaction to dentistry. *J. Dent. Child.* **42,** 290–2.

Thrash W. J., Marr J. N., Boone S. E. (1982) Continuous self-monitoring of discomfort in the dental chair and feedback to the dentist. *J. Behav. Assessment* **4,** 273–84.

Venham L. L. (1979) The effect of mother's presence on child's responses to dental treatment. *J. Dent. Child.* **46,** 219–25.

Weinstein P., Nathan J. (1988) The challenge of fearful and phobic children. In *The Dental Clinics of North America* (Rubin J.G., Kaplan A., eds). **32,** 667–92.

Wright G. L., Alpern G. D., Leake J. L. (1973) The modifiability of maternal anxiety as it relates to children's co-operative dental behaviour. *J. Dent. Child.* **40,** 265–71.

Chapter 5

Pain

The possibility that a visit to the dentist will be a painful one is an important consideration for many patients. It is often cited as a reason for both avoidance and anxiety. Nor is it an unrealistic concern: depending on how it is measured, up to 77% of patients report that they feel some pain during their visit (Klepac et al., 1980a). However, it seems that some dentists do not appreciate the importance of this factor for patients. In one survey of 20 dentists, 16 denied that their patients experienced any pain. One dentist stated: 'Only once in every five years do I have a patient who has pain' (Dangott et al., 1978). The reason for this discrepancy is not clear, but it may be partly because some dentists assume that modern analgesics and technical equipment are adequate to eliminate pain completely.

The aim of this chapter is to explore some of the research on pain and pain relief. The first section outlines some of the basic ideas behind modern theories of pain. Research in this area is complicated by the problem that there are many factors which influence both how much pain a person feels and how much pain a person reports. Ways of measuring pain are considered in the second section. Consideration of these ideas is important for the understanding of psychological approaches to pain relief, which are considered in the third part of the chapter.

Taken together, these studies demonstrate the fallacy of the distinction which is often made between the mind and the body, between anatomy, biochemistry and physiology on the one hand and psychology and sociology on the other. While this distinction between the biological and the behavioural sciences has certain advantages, it can lead to some misleading assumptions. It is certainly not a useful approach where pain is concerned.

The experience of pain

The problem with taking a purely biological approach to pain is that it does not provide an adequate explanation for many observations. One assumption which follows from this approach is that the magnitude of an injury should show a close correspondence with the amount of pain experienced. While this may often be the case, there are so many exceptions to the rule that it must be seen as an oversimplification. Beecher (1946) made some critical observations during World War II while he was treating soldiers wounded in battle. To his surprise, he found that many soldiers (around 60%) who had been severely wounded reported only slight pain or even no pain at all. During his civilian practice, where patients had received similar injuries because of surgery, virtually all had requested analgesics.

At first, Beecher considered the possibility that the soldiers were in fact feeling much pain but were unwilling to report it, perhaps because this would be inconsistent with their views of themselves as stoic and uncomplaining. However, this did not seem to be an adequate explanation because the soldiers did complain loudly about the relatively slight pain involved in injections. Beecher concluded that it was not necessarily the magnitude of an injury which was significant but, rather, the circumstances in which it occurred. In fact, readers who have participated in sports may have had less traumatic but similar experiences: athletes sometimes find that although they sustained an injury during a game they did not notice it until the competition had finished. Similar surprises can be found in dentistry. One would expect, for example, that larger gauges of needles used for injections would result in more pain than smaller gauges, yet when Fuller et al. (1979) tested this, no differences in the amount of pain felt with 25G, 27G or 30G needles could be found.

The puzzle of these observations is complicated further by observations about when pain occurs. From a biological view, no pain would be expected when there is no injury, and every injury should result in pain. However there are reports of quite severe injuries being suffered with little pain, as in some religious ceremonies in India where large steel hooks are inserted in the back muscles. At the height of the ceremony, the participants are suspended by these hooks but they seem to tolerate these injuries with little discomfort (Kosambi, 1967). Conversely, there are occasions when people experience pain without recent injury, as in phantom limb pain. Patients who have a limb amputated sometimes complain of pain in the leg or arm which has been removed—pain that is persistent, long-term and difficult to relieve (Simmel, 1962). Pain in paraplegic patients can be particularly disturbing. Paraplegia refers to a total loss of sensation and motor activity after damage to the spinal cord. This pain can occur even when the cord is totally transected (Melzack and Loeser, 1978).

Gate Theory

Observations such as these render purely anatomical and physiological explanations of pain unsatisfactory and several theories have been put forward to explain them. Perhaps the most successful is Melzack and Wall's Gate Theory (1982). Briefly, they suggest that the experience of pain involves not only physical sensations from an injury but also emotional and evaluative reactions to these sensations. They argue that signals from an injured site run to the dorsal horn of the spinal cord which acts like a kind of gate between peripheral fibres and the brain. The gate is opened (i.e. the dorsal horn cells are excited) by small fibres from the site of the stimulation and closed by other large inhibitory fibres from the same site.

These do not provide the only influences on the gate: it is also affected by fibres from the brainstem reticular formation which serve to excite or inhibit the dorsal horn cells. Reticular formations are also affected by cortical activity, so that past experiences, anxiety, attention and the meaning of the situation influence the opening and closing of the gate. A patient who has had painful dental experiences in the past or who expects much pain could actually experience more discomfort.

Components of pain
Melzack and Wall make a distinction between three components which contribute to the experience of pain. The first component is the *sensory–discriminative*, which determines the perceptual information received by the individual. Such information includes the location, magnitude and timing of the stimulus. The second is the *affective–motivational* component, which provides the motivation to act as a result of this information. The third *cognitive–evaluative* component is affected by past experiences and expectations. Taken together, these interact to determine how much distress a person feels and how he or she will react to the distress.

Melzack and Wall use this model to account for many of the above observations. They argue, for example, that the sudden loss of a limb through amputation removes not only the excitatory fibres running from the injury but also the inhibitory ones, so that the gate may remain permanently open. This could explain why people who have phantom limb pain may feel the discomfort involved in the injury that led to the amputation rather than the amputation itself. It also accounts for why limb loss through leprosy, where the process is much more gradual, does not lead to phantom limb pain. For the World War II soldiers seen by Beecher, being injured on the battlefield had positive connotations, in that it meant that they would be rested away from the fighting and most unlikely to be killed. For the civilian patients, a similar operation was life-threatening and a disruption to their normal routine.

Minimal tissue damage can cause severe pain if the signals from the brain open the gate wider than usual. Patients could be very sensitive to any slight tissue damage if they were very anxious or fearful of it. What might seem to be painless to one patient may be very painful to another. Gate Theory can be used to explain some data collected by Burstein and Burstein (1979) on dental patients' responses to injections. Before the treatment, they asked patients to indicate how much pain they had experienced from injections in the past and how much they expected on this occasion. After treatment the patients were again interviewed, this time being asked how much pain they had actually experienced. Gate theory would predict significant correlations between these measures and this is what the Bursteins found: memory and actual experience correlated 0.52, expectation and experience 0.80.

Implications of gate theory

Psychogenic versus somatogenic pain
The important point here is that psychological, physiological and situational factors interact to produce what a person experiences. For the present purposes, this has three important implications. One involves the traditional distinction between somatogenic and psychogenic pain. Somatogenic pain refers to pain which has a describable objective basis, such as a bone fracture or appendicitis. A pain is said to be psychogenic if there is no discernible tissue damage: the idea here is that the pain's aetiology can be found in the psychological and not the physical state of the patient. According to this approach, pain is *either* psychogenic *or* somatogenic. Gate Theory suggests a somewhat different approach, as represented in Fig. 5.1. Here, every pain is considered to have *both* psychogenic *and* somatogenic components, although one or the other may predominate for any individual in a particular situation (Dworkin et al., 1978).

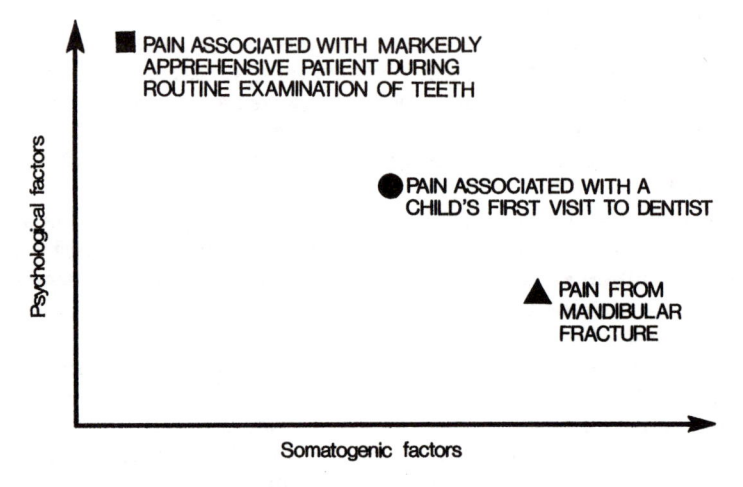

Figure 5.1 According to gate theory, all pain has both psychogenic and somatogenic influences, although one or the other may predominate. From Dworkin et al. (1978), with permission.

Previous learning
A second implication of Gate Theory is that the experience of pain depends, in part, on previous learning. This was demonstrated long ago by Pavlov during his work on classical conditioning. Normally, dogs react strongly when an electric shock is applied to one of their paws. Pavlov was able to show that they could be taught to react with apparent pleasure if he consistently presented food after each shock. The dogs would salivate and wag their tails each time they were shocked, showing no aversive reactions. What was once painful came to be a positive event—a signal that food was about to be given. Interestingly, when Pavlov changed the site of the shock from one paw to another it again elicited a violent response, indicating that the learning was locally determined to some extent.

It seems that learning about pain also occurs in humans. Many doctors have noted that reactions to painful stimuli often 'run in families'—parents and their children seem to react in similar ways—but it is difficult to distinguish between biological and environmental influences. Perhaps children react like their parents because they are genetically similar or because their parents 'teach' them to react in certain ways, or both.

Research
A third implication of gate theory concerns research. Since the meaning of a situation has such an important influence on pain, the results of experiments on pain relief undertaken in the laboratory may not apply to the clinical situation. Laboratory-induced pain differs from clinically induced pain in several ways. It is short-lived and can be stopped on request, but clinical pain can be persistent, beyond the patient's control and often accompanied by high levels of anxiety. In the laboratory, pain is induced by stimuli which are novel (e.g. electric shocks, heat or cold water) whereas patients often have prior experience with clinical pain, either directly or through observations of others' reactions. Where attempts have been made to predict postoperative need for analgesics, patients react differently in the laboratory than they do on a hospital ward (Parbrook et al., 1973). Another finding which suggests that the two types of pain are different is that morphine, which is very effective for reducing pain for clinical patients, is often ineffective in reducing laboratory-induced pain.

Even when the kind of pain induced in a laboratory closely approximates clinical pain, caution is required. One popular method used in laboratory studies of dental pain is tooth shock: an electric current is passed into an incisor. In a test of the effects of the clinical setting on responses to this painful stimulus, Dworkin and Chen (1982) administered tooth shock to two groups of volunteers. Half of them were given the shocks in a laboratory setting, while for the other half they were given in a dentist's surgery by someone who identified himself as a dentist. All of the volunteers were given an ascending series of shocks: their task was to indicate when they first began to feel the shocks (sensation threshold), when the shocks first became painful (pain threshold) and when they could tolerate no more (pain tolerance). On all three measures, those given tooth shock in the dentist's surgery reported more pain. They reached the sensation and pain thresholds at lower amperages and wanted the study to terminate earlier. Thus, the different contexts of a laboratory and a dentist's office affected the amount of pain experienced, even though the stimulus was the same. For all these reasons, it is important that techniques for pain relief which have proved successful in the laboratory should be validated in clinical settings before they can be recommended with any confidence.

Acute versus chronic pain

The distinction between acute and chronic pain is somewhat arbitrary: pain of recent onset is generally termed acute, but if it persists for several months it is termed chronic. Acute pain is associated with heightened autonomic arousal (e.g. increases in heart rate, blood pressure and striated muscle tone), but patients with chronic pain show habituation of autonomic signs.

From a practical point of view, acute and chronic pain have different psychological consequences. Anxiety is a common response to acute pain and the autonomic signs are consistent with the 'fight or flight' response. Chronic pain (such as that found in temporomandibular joint (TMJ) disorder patients, see Chapter 6) has more lasting effects. Depression is frequent and there can be severe curtailment of lifestyle as patients guard against exacerbating discomfort. This can result in a vicious circle: as individuals become more careful about movements their attention becomes increasingly focused on their bodily sensations. This in turn makes movement increasingly painful. These problems are reflected by what patients say to themselves. Phillips (1989) found that chronic pain patients would often dwell upon their discomfort (e.g. 'I wonder if they will ever find a cure for my pain?') and its effects (e.g. 'How am I going to concentrate with this awful pain?'). In such instances pain can come to dominate a person, resulting in severe incapacity.

Measuring pain

Before discussing psychological interventions, it is first necessary to consider how pain could be measured. The basic problem here (as in the measurement of anxiety) is that pain is a private experience, one that cannot be seen or felt by anyone else. Thus, some kind of indirect method must be used. Physiological, self-report and behavioural methods are three possibilities.

Physiological measures

Several physiological indices of acute stress have been employed. The level of corticosteroids in the blood, heart rate, respiration rate and the amount of perspiration are some measures. The amount of perspiration is measured by the galvanic skin response: the resistance between two electrodes placed a set distance apart on the skin. The palmar sweat index concerns the number of open sweat glands: a piece of sticky tape is placed over a finger and then this is removed and examined under a microscope. While there is no reason to believe that these physiological measures are any less valid than those listed below, it is important to point out that there is often a low correlation between different physiological measures (Leiderman and Shapiro, 1965).

Self-report measures

The most frequently used self-report method is some version of a 10-cm line with extremes marked at either end (such as 'the pain is as bad as it could be' and 'I have no pain'). This is called the Visual Analogue Scale or VAS. Patients are asked to place an 'x' somewhere between the extremes indicating the degree of pain they experience. Then it is a simple procedure to measure the distance from one end of the scale to give a quantitative score (Scott and Huskisson, 1976). This measure of severity is intended to include the sensory, affective and evaluative components of pain.

Those who have used this technique have worked on the assumption that, because the scale is marked privately, it provides an accurate indication of patients' feelings, being relatively unaffected by what they believe should be expressed to others. However, it is not clear how valid this assumption is. Different cultural groups, for example, express their pain differently, with some reporting more than others. People with a Northern European background tend to express their pain less readily than those from Latin countries (Zola, 1966). Even if the patient fills out the scale unobserved, such differences could be expected to be still operating. Personality characteristics are also associated with how much pain a person reports, with some more willing than others to express discomfort.

The McGill Pain Questionnaire

The McGill Pain Questionnaire or MPQ (Melzack, 1975) was designed to measure severity of pain along the three dimensions suggested by Gate Theory. The patient is asked to choose adjectives from a total of 20 lists which best describe the pain. Some lists refer to sensory aspects, others to the affective and evaluative ones, as shown in Table 5.1. Within each list the adjectives are rank ordered such that a choice of, say, 'pounding' would be given a higher score than 'flickering' or 'quivering'. The amount of pain a person feels can be quantified by both the number of adjectives chosen and the weighting given to each one. Furthermore, some idea of the relative importance of each of the three dimensions can be gained.

Some examples of how different groups of patients respond to the questionnaire are also shown in Table 5.1. Many dental patients describe toothache as 'throbbing' on a sensory list, as 'sickening' on the affective and 'annoying' on the evaluative (Dubuisson and Melzack, 1976). By contrast, childbirth is often called 'pounding', 'exhausting' and 'intense' (Melzack et al., 1981). Van Buren and Kleinknecht (1979) asked patients

Table 5.1 Some of the list of adjectives from the Melzack pain questionnaire. Patients are asked to choose those words which best describe their pain

Sensory	Affective		Evaluative
Flickering	Sickening†	Tiring	Annoying†
Quivering	Suffocating	Exhausting*	Troublesome
Pulsing			Miserable
Throbbing†			Intense*
Beating			Unbearable
Pounding*			

*Words often chosen by women to describe labour; †words often chosen by patients to describe toothache.
From Dworkin et al. (1978), with permission.

who had a tooth extracted to fill out the questionnaire on three occasions—the evening after the extraction and on the next 2 days. They found that the sensory and evaluative components showed a decrease in intensity, but the affective component remained about the same.

This is a most interesting approach to pain measurement and is becoming increasingly popular. Part of its attraction is that it might be possible to tailor pain-relief techniques to particular individuals. A patient who scores highly on the sensory dimension might be given a different kind of treatment than one whose pain is mainly affective. It might also be possible to use the results in making a diagnosis. Work by Grushka and Sessle (1984) suggests that the MPQ could be used to distinguish pain originating from a reversibly inflamed tooth pulp and pain from an irreversibly inflamed or necrotic pulp. Thus MPQ results could be useful to the clinician if there is uncertainty about the vitality of the tooth. However such an approach is in its infancy and would benefit from further study.

Validity
The obvious way to test the validity of these self-report methods is to provide analgesics and then look for differences in pain reports. Generally, self-reports do show a decrease in pain after analgesic administration. Unfortunately, comparisons between the subjective pain-rating scales have shown that they do not correlate particularly well, indicating that they are measuring somewhat different aspects of the pain experience (Reading, 1980).

Behavioural measures

Non-verbal signs
Another kind of approach to measurement relies upon the behaviour of the patient. Non-verbal signs such as grimacing or tightening of the muscles during a dental procedure could indicate pain. Darwin suggested that facial expressions are largely genetically determined, and people from different cultures throughout the world show similar expressions for anger, fear, pain and so on (Ekman, 1973).

There is some interesting work on the possibility that there is a reciprocal relationship between experienced pain and facial expressiveness. That is, people may use their expressions to indicate to others and to *themselves* how much pain they feel. There are two studies of interest here, both of which involved giving electric shocks. Kleck et al. (1976) were interested in how people would react if they knew they were being watched as compared to when they believed they were alone. In our culture many people believe that they should not exhibit too much distress when others are present, so Kleck et al. hypothesized that people who believed themselves to be observed would show fewer indications of pain than those who believed themselves alone.

Everyone was videotaped so that their expressions could be monitored. As predicted, those who knew they were being watched showed less distress than those who believed themselves alone, indicating that expressiveness is open to social influence. However, this was only half the story. The people in the experiment were also asked to rate the painfulness of the shocks, and their skin conductance was measured. Those who were told that they would be observed gave lower pain ratings and were less physiologically aroused. Skin conductance is not easily brought under control, so there was little chance of 'faking' on this measure. In other words, being observed seemed to result in less pain.

The question is, why did this occur? Perhaps the effects of being observed were indirect. Being observed affected expressiveness. It seems possible that those in the observed condition were using kinesthetic feedback from their own expressions as cues to help them judge just how painful the electric shocks were. In order to test this possibility, Lanzetta et al. (1976) first gave electric shocks to everyone in their study, while taking a measure of skin conductance. This provided baseline data. Then, half were instructed to reveal their discomfort through exaggerated facial expressions, while the other half were asked to hide their feelings. Some of the results are shown in Fig. 5.2. At both high and low shock levels, the 'reveal' group were more physiologically aroused than the 'hide' group, indicating that they felt more pain. Thus, it seems that facial expressiveness is used as a kind of feedback indicating how much pain is experienced.

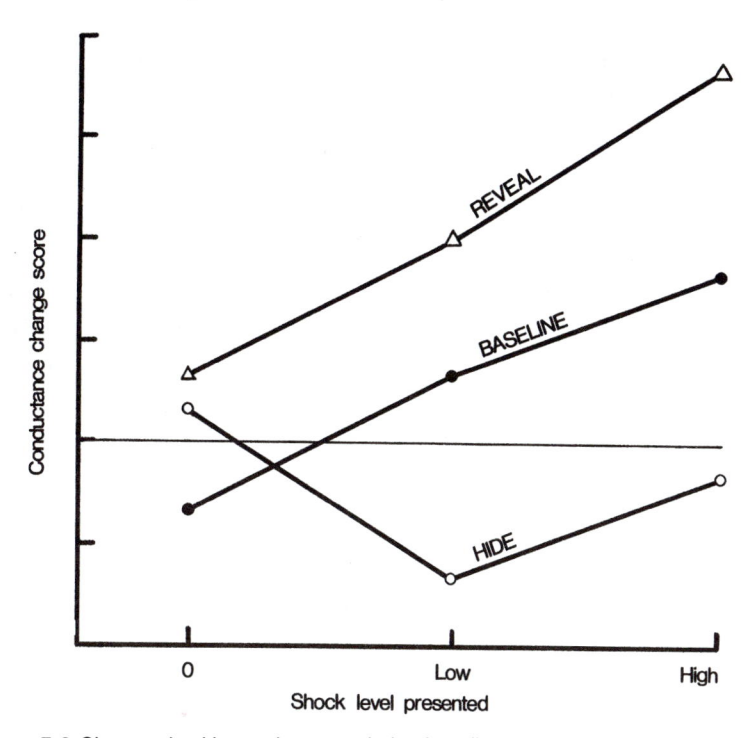

Figure 5.2 Changes in skin conductance during baseline measures and when those in the experiment were instructed either to 'reveal' or 'hide' their pain. From Lanzetta et al. (1976), with permission.

Requests for analgesics

Instead of looking for non-verbal signs of pain, patients' requests for analgesics could be monitored. This might provide an objective measure of subjective feelings. Unfortunately, there are problems here too, since requests for analgesics seem to be influenced by cultural and personality factors. This problem was encountered earlier when pain rating scales were discussed. The Eysenck Personality Inventory (EPI) (Eysenck, 1967) has been used in some studies on this topic. The introversion–extroversion scale of the EPI is designed to measure the extent to which an individual is outgoing, sociable and impulsive. It seems that extroverts are more likely to voice their feelings about pain and make requests for pain-relievers than are introverts (Bond, 1980).

Staff responses

An alternative approach would be to monitor the amount of analgesic given by staff. Nurses, for example, could be expected to be very competent in recognizing the signs due to their wide experience. Bond and Pilowski (1966) took self-report measures of pain using 10-cm scales, and then monitored patients' requests for analgesics and the responses of the nursing staff. They found that the perception of pain did not always result in a request for medication, requests when made did not always lead to administration by staff and the strength of the medication when it was given was not proportional to pain levels. The sex of the patient seemed particularly relevant (Table 5.2). Nursing staff were much more likely to take the initiative with female patients in administering analgesics and more likely to refuse requests from male patients. The suggestion is that cultural expectations were operating: the nurses may have believed that men should be able to tolerate more pain than women.

Table 5.2 Pattern of administration of analgesic drugs to men and women in radiotherapy wards: drugs requested and given during 1 week

	Men	Women
Number of patients	15	12
Number of occasions drugs given at patient's request	23	28
Number of occasions drugs given on initiative of nurses	1	22
Number of occasions on which nurses refused patient's request for drugs	18	0

From Bond (1979), with permission.

Impact on lifestyle

This type of measure is more suited to the effects of chronic than acute pain. For the general dental practitioner it could form part of the assessment for patients with TMJ problems. As mentioned earlier in the chapter, chronic discomfort can pervade a person's lifestyle, such that activity is restricted and attention is almost permanently focused on the pain. Marital satisfaction, social interactions, recreational activities and employment could all be affected (Pearce and Erskine, 1989). The Sickness

Impact Profile (Bergner and Bobbitt, 1981) provides scores on several dimensions, including emotions, work, sleep, eating and recreation.

These difficulties with the measurement of pain illustrate the complexity of the phenomenon. Since pain itself is open to so many influences it is not surprising that measuring techniques are similarly affected. But it does present problems for pain control research. One important problem concerns the finding that physiological, self-report and behavioural indices of pain do not always correlate with each other. As in the measurement of anxiety, it may be important to consider all three aspects when testing the efficacy of a technique for relieving pain.

Alleviating pain

According to Gate Theory, there are three components which contribute to the experience of pain: the sensory–discriminative, the affective–motivational and the cognitive–evaluative. Modification of any of these would be expected to reduce the distress felt by a patient. The techniques outlined below are grouped under these three headings, although it should be said that some methods, such as relaxation and hypnosis, may be operating on more than one component at the same time. Here, the primary concern is with acute pain, as might be experienced in the dental surgery due to restorations or extractions. Chronic pain, such as that found in the TMJ pain dysfunction syndrome, presents different problems which may require different solutions, as considered in the next chapter.

Pain and anxiety

The contribution that pain makes to anxiety is, as discussed in Chapter 3, not altogether clear. It seems most useful to consider pain and anxiety as interdependent, such that one can lead to the other. There is some evidence that dentally anxious patients are more sensitive to dental pain than non-anxious patients (Klepac et al., 1980b). When Lautch (1971) attempted to find ways of distinguishing between phobic and non-phobic patients, he found that phobic patients had a pain threshold level some 28% below the non-phobics. While it is not possible to say that increased sensitivity *causes* anxiety, it seems that there is an association between the two.

Thus it is no coincidence that some of the techniques discussed below have been encountered by the reader before in the previous chapter on relieving anxiety. Since anxiety is one of the contributing factors to pain and pain to anxiety, a reduction in one should lead to a reduction in the other. Thus a frightened patient may benefit from these methods both by a decrease in distress due to anxiety and by a decrease in distress due to pain.

The sensory–discriminative component

There are several techniques which affect this component of pain. The aim of surgical procedures is to destroy neural pathways which carry impulses from the injured site. Cutting can be done peripherally or centrally: cordotomy, for example, involves cutting the spinal cord. Pharmacological techniques provide short-term relief. Novocain works by blocking nerve conduction, while morphine seems to be effective because it is similar to enkephalins—endogenous narcotic-like substances.

The placebo effect

In studies on pain relief it is important to include a group of people who do not receive the active treatment but instead an equally plausible alternative. This is to control for placebo effects, which are those effects of a procedure that are not due to the treatment itself, but rather to the circumstances surrounding it. These include the warmth and enthusiasm of the therapist, the patient's hopes and expectations that he or she will get better and the mechanics of administering the treatment (e.g. an injection or the taking of pills). Placebo effects have been shown in most areas of patient care, such as surgery, psychotherapy and the alleviation of pain (Shapiro and Morris, 1978). Figure 5.3, for example, shows the percentage of cancer patients reporting at least 50% pain relief from morphine or saline solution. There was a substantial effect from saline solution alone and the time–effect curve mimicked that of morphine (Houde et al., 1960). If there were no control groups in pain relief studies any decreases in pain could be due to circumstances such as the

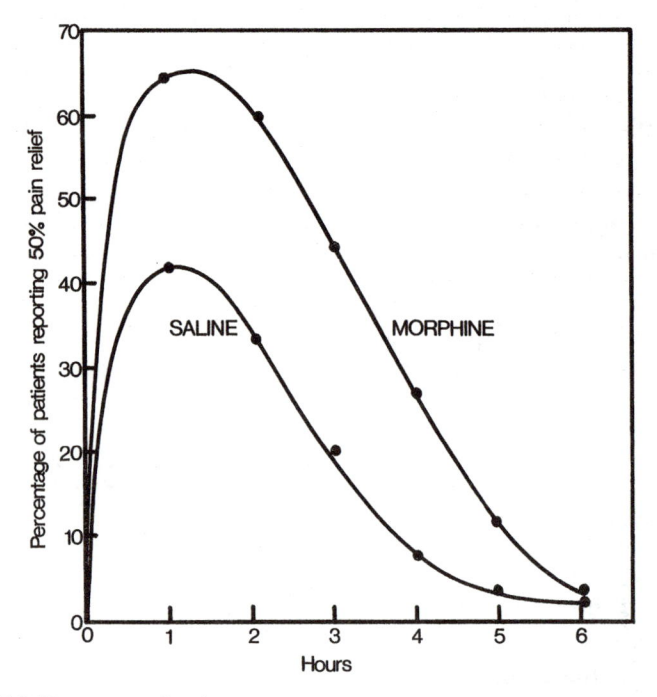

Figure 5.3 Percentage of patients reporting at least 50% pain relief over a 6-h period from 10 mg morphine sulphate or sterile saline. From Houde et al. (1960), with permission.

attention given to the patients or simply the suggestion that the treatment will be effective.

How do placebos work?
Although the results shown in Fig. 5.3 are not unusual, they are often misinterpreted. Many people believe that the placebo effect occurs for most people most of the time. This is not the case. On average, about 35% of patients obtain relief, but this varies from 0 to 100% depending on the disease and situational factors such as the patients' and dentists' beliefs about the efficacy of treatment. Personality traits and demographic characteristics (such as age and sex) are not consistently related to whether an individual responds to a placebo.

When placebos are effective, though, what processes are involved? One theory relies on classical conditioning (see Chapter 3). In some studies by Pavlov, dogs were given morphine and, as in the case of food and salivation, some of the animals came to show a response to morphine before they were given an injection. The suggestion is that in humans the placebo effect operates in a similar way: patients feel better because this is a conditioned response to taking medication.

Another possibility has to do with selective attention. In most illnesses, the amount of discomfort varies, so a patient will feel better at some times than at others. This is certainly true of the discomfort after an extraction. Placebo effects could occur if patients became more aware of the times they did feel better and paid less attention to the times when they felt unwell. Yet another suggestion is that patients may come to interpret their sensations as less unpleasant following a dentist's advice. Gate Theory postulates that the experience of pain is enhanced by anxiety, such that the gate in the dorsal horn is opened by fear. When a dentist says that a pain reliever will reduce discomfort after an extraction—implying that discomfort is to be expected and will respond to medication—anxiety could decrease and the gate close.

A more recent suggestion is that placebos work through the release of endorphins (endogenous morphine-like substances) into the body. This suggestion has been tested by the administration of naloxone, an opiate antagonist which blocks the opiate receptor sites. If when naloxone is given the placebo effect is no longer found, this would provide evidence for a link between endorphins and placebos. Levine et al. (1978) studied patients whose impacted wisdom teeth were to be removed. Two hours after surgery all patients were given a placebo and then, after a further hour, either placebo or naloxone. As expected, those patients who were given naloxone reported greater pain than did those given a placebo. Although this study suggests that the analgesic effect of placebos is based on endorphins, it does not answer the interesting question of how the message 'Take this, it will make you feel better' from a trusted dentist is translated into the release of endorphins.

The affective–motivation component

This component refers to the ways in which people react to the sensory information they receive. They could react with much distress if the information was taken as a threat to their well-being, a threat which could not be overcome or tolerated. If the information could be considered more neutrally, without affective connotations, the patient might feel that he or she could cope with the situation in some way. The aim would be to encourage the latter kind of reaction while reducing the former. In this section two techniques are discussed which have been shown to be useful in this way. First, the idea of distraction is explored and second, the possibility of giving the patient some control over the dentist's behaviour is considered.

Distraction
The idea behind the use of distraction is that patients can be provided with ways of coping with their experiences. Instead of dwelling on the sensory input, they can shift their attention away to some other kind of stimulus. One of the earlier studies in this area involved what is called audioanalgesia. Gardner and Licklinder (1959) reasoned that one of the causes of pain and anxiety in dental patients was the grinding noise of the drill. The noise was thought to raise apprehension and increase tension. They arranged for their patients to have some means of masking this noise, being given a choice of white noise (a hissing sound containing a wide range of frequencies) or music. The patients could also control the volume level. In a series of 387 patients, all of whom received cavity preparations and all of whom had previously required gas or local anaesthetic, completely effective analgesia was found for 63%. Adequate analgesia was produced in 25%, while for only 12% was the technique not successful. This method was also effective in reducing pain during extractions.

Some other reports of audioanalgesia have supported this technique, though rarely with such significant results. There is some evidence that it is important that patients should be told that the white noise or music will be effective in reducing their pain. Without this suggestion the method may not be successful (Melzack et al., 1963). Whereas Gardner and Licklinder suggested that audioanalgesia works by masking the noise of the drill, it seems more likely that it is effective because it distracts the patient's attention away from the dentist's drilling and towards the white noise or music.

Another method for distracting patients is to ask them to perform some kind of mental task during treatment. It may be particularly useful to encourage the imagination of pleasant and refreshing scenes rather than the performance of repetitious and dull tasks. Horan et al. (1976), for example, asked patients to listen to a tape-recording describing such relaxing scenes as walking through a lush meadow and swimming in a clear blue lake. In order to control for any placebo effects of the listening to the tape and to test the efficacy of this kind of distraction over others, the patients were also asked to listen to another tape. This tape listed a series of two-digit numbers every 15 s and the patients' task was to imagine these numerals on a plain piece of white cardboard. On a self-report measure of distress, encouragement to imagine the pleasant scenes was the more effective technique, perhaps because it was more likely to capture the patient's attention.

It seems that many patients have learned to use such distraction techniques without a dentist's intervention. They might concentrate on some other part of the body or on some object in the surgery. Thus, it might be useful to provide objects in the surgery which all patients could use to distract themselves, even if they are not showing any overt signs of pain. Hanging an interesting painting where they can see it while the dentist is working, for example, or giving them a choice of music to listen to could provide useful distractions.

Besides distraction, there are other cognitive techniques which can be used to change the emotional qualities of pain. There are indications that if patients can be encouraged to re-interpret the sensations they feel then pain may be reduced. For example, Langer et al. (1975) asked the surgical patients in their study to try interpret the pain they felt as optimistically as possible. They were asked to consider it as an indication that they were getting better and that it signalled an eventual improvement in their health. These and other instructions had positive effects on their recovery from the operations. As rated by nurses, for example, these patients showed less anxiety and a greater ability to cope with the post-operative period.

Enhancing control
One reason why distraction and the other cognitive strategies might be helpful is that they provide patients with some degree of control over their feelings. The idea that giving patients control over their dentists' behaviour through some kind of stop signal has been given consistent support (Thompson, 1981). It should be pointed out that control in the sense meant here does not mean the possibility of avoiding the situation but rather the ability to influence the manner of experiencing it.

Wardle (1982) describes how she used a stop signal to reduce pain. All patients were attending a dentist for routine care, mostly fillings. Some patients were shown a stop signal—the raising of an arm—and were told that they could use it as often as they needed, whenever they wanted a rest. The dentist said that he wished them to use it at least once. For another group of patients the dentist went about his work as usual. When the patients were interviewed after the appointment, 50% of the patients given routine care reported some pain, but only 15% of those who had been told about the stop signal. In another study (Thrash et al., 1982a), significant reductions in pain and discomfort due to the injection were found. Patients were given buttons to push which lit green (signalling relative comfort), yellow (some discomfort) and red (considerable discomfort) lights. They were told that the dentist would stop when the red light was on. Whatever the stop signal, it seems particularly important that the dentist should respond quickly and unambiguously to a patient's discomfort (Thrash et al., 1982b).

The cognitive–evaluative component

This component is primarily concerned with an evaluation of the severity of the sensory input. Is the experience only annoying or is it intense or even unbearable? Gate Theory indicates that patients' *expectations* about the intensity of the stimulus they will experience are very important in this respect. It has been argued that part of the difficulty that patients face in undergoing dental procedures is the way that professional dental care has come to be labelled as 'painful', so that any intense stimulation experienced in the dentist's chair is taken to be pain. Some research on this contention is discussed below, along with two further methods which seek to alter expectations about pain in dentistry, hypnosis and preparing the patient for treatment.

The word 'pain'
Several dentists have suggested that this word should be avoided whenever possible, lest the patient come to label (and feel) dental procedures as painful. In general, it is better to avoid emotive words when describing the effects of a dental procedure to a patient; for example, to use the word 'restore' rather than 'drill' (Jan, 1964). It may often be possible to provide labels which do not have emotional connotations. Neiberger (1978) reports some positive results using this approach with children who were visiting the dentist to have their teeth cleaned. They were all greeted by the words 'Hello. How are you? Today we are going to clean your teeth with a magic toothbrush and toothpaste.' The number of children who co-operated with the dentist and who laughed during the cleaning was noted. Half-way through the cleaning the dentist then added: 'When I brush your teeth it will tickle and make you laugh', a comment which seemed to have an important effect on the children's behaviour.

Before this second statement, 40% of the children showed some resistance, but only 4% afterwards. Seventy-four per cent started to laugh during the second half of the appointment, compared to only 7% beforehand. Using the word 'tickle' as a label for the sensations seemed to make the cleaning enjoyable rather than distressing. One problem with this study is that the children may have become more co-operative simply because they found the cleaning to be less distressing than they expected or simply because they became more used to it as the appointment progressed. It would have been better to have conducted the experiment on two groups of children, one group who were told that the cleaning would tickle and one group who were not told this.

Hypnosis
Like many other complex skills, hypnosis requires some considerable training and both patients and therapists become more proficient with practice. Although there are few well controlled studies on hypnosis in dentisty (Kent, 1986), many case studies have indicated that much of the discomfort and anxiety associated with dental care can be alleviated. The general aim of hypnosis is to help patients achieve a sense of calm well-being and a belief that they can cope with the stress of the situation (Smith, 1987).

There are a number of induction techniques, but their success seems to depend on the patient's motivation and trust in the hypnotherapist. Generally, the patient is asked to focus attention on one object, concentrating on it completely without allowing other thoughts to intrude. Coe

(1980), for example, describes how he uses a pendulum, held by the patient, in order to induce concentration and openness to suggestion:

> I want you to hold this little bob just the way I do. (Demonstrate the proper way to hold the thread.) That's it, just hold it so you can sit there comfortably and relax. Now I want you to take the attitude just for a moment or so, that that little bob is the only thing of importance to you. That's it, just focus your gaze on it, and begin trying to discover all you can about it. (It is helpful if the bob has designs, colors, or other irregularities on it.) That's it, look at it carefully, trace all around its outline, notice any geometric shapes that may be on it, like circles—squares—perhaps you can even find rectangles if you look carefully. Just try to learn everything you can about that little bob, think of it as a new and different experience, something unique, something you would like to know everything about. Notice its colors—notice how this varies from spot to spot, and how it changes—as you become more interested in the bob, you notice that in fact it becomes more the center of your attention. Your vision narrows, things in the side of your vision tend to grey out, to become less important. The bob in fact becomes the center of your attention—now watch it very closely, because in a moment it is going to begin doing something—it will begin moving back and forth, back and forth, back and forth (p. 449).

Suggestions which are easy to follow are given first (e.g. that their attention on the pendulum has caused their eyes to become tired and the eyelids heavy). Relaxation plays an important part, with suggestions that arms and legs are becoming heavier and more relaxed. Often, patients are asked to count backwards from 10 or from 20, becoming more relaxed with each number.

When hypnotized, the patient is more open to the therapist's suggestions than in the 'waking' state. Suggestions aimed at lessening such problems as pain or anxiety are more likely to be accepted. The hypnotized person is able to listen and speak to the therapist and remains aware of who he is and what is going on around him. Patients will also reject any suggestions they find distasteful or unacceptable, so there is no question that the hypnotist controls patients against their will. Suggestions can be made in the hypnotic state to which patients can respond later, when they have 'awoken'—a phenomenon known as 'post-hypnotic suggestion'. In addition, subjects can be shown how to hypnotize themselves. Therapists regard this self-hypnosis, also known as 'auto-hypnosis', as very useful because individuals can attain a relaxed state quickly in the absence of the hypnotist.

A trance state?
Although hypnosis was popular in the 19th century, it was until very recently considered with much scepticism. Part of the reason for this lack of acceptance was the problem of knowing what a hypnotic state might be. Many hypnotists characterize it as a 'trance state'—a unique form of consciousness where some critical faculties are suspended—but it is difficult to distinguish hypnotized people from those who have been coached to behave in certain ways. Many of the feats ascribed to hypnosis can be attained by most people when in the waking state. For example, stage hypnotists often suggest that a person will become rigid,

so much so that he will be able to support himself with the neck on the edge of one chair and the heels on the edge of another. This looks impressive but, in fact, it can be accomplished by most fit people.

Susceptibility and pain relief
A more profitable approach has involved the investigation of susceptibility, defined as the degree to which a person is 'able to enter into hypnosis and become involved in its characteristic behaviour' (Engstrom, 1976). Several scales have been developed to test for susceptibility, such as the Stanford Hypnotic Susceptibility Scale (Weitzenhoffer and Hilgard, 1959). Several short tests are used, such as the willingness to fall backwards into the hypnotist's arms. There are some indications that the level of susceptibility is important because it is associated with the amount of pain relief a person will experience under hypnosis. As shown in Fig. 5.4 people with high susceptibility receive more pain relief than those with low susceptibility (Hilgard, 1975).

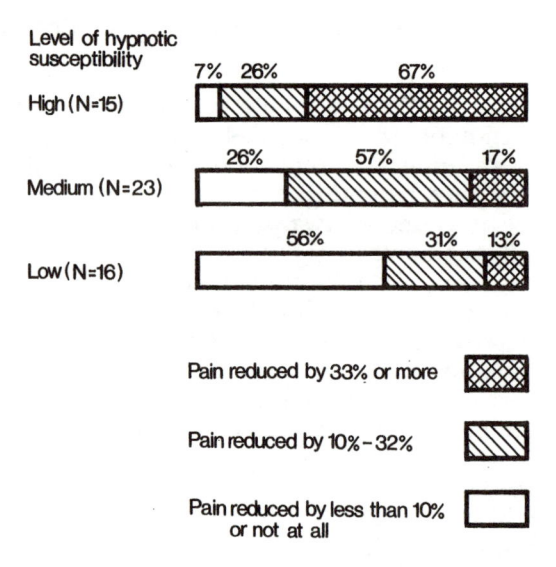

Figure 5.4 People with low susceptibility to hypnosis often experience less pain relief than people with high susceptibility. From Hilgard (1975), with permission.

Anxiety
As mentioned earlier, hypnosis can also be used to relieve anxiety, a state which can reduce the effectiveness of analgesics. This is illustrated by the following case study (Fier, 1980):

> A twelve-year-old girl, named Mary, came to see me for routine dental care. Her general health was fine, but she reported having had a 'bad' experience in a dental office when she was 6 or 7 years old. She wouldn't tell me very much about it, and since her parents weren't present during treatment, no further information could be obtained. On further questioning Mary would only say that this dentist hurt her and nothing more. When she spoke of this

experience she began shaking and was visibly upset. On her first visit Mary requested 'gas', since she had experienced it before. We began analgesia and routine excavation, but we had to stop and temporize the teeth. We couldn't find a comfortable level of analgesia for her. As soon as she relaxed, she'd pass into an excitement stage. The stage of analgesia for Mary was almost non-existent. During her next visit, I began her hypnotic induction through visual fixation, deep breathing, and counting exercises. Using the technique of taking the patient in and out of a trance quickly and repeatedly, along with other suggestions, I was able to deepen her level of relaxation. At this point Mary's shaking stopped. Using 'eraser technique' (as a schoolteacher erases a blackboard) I facilitated Mary 'erasing' from her memory the past experience that had caused her so much discomfort. With some other suggestions, we were able to help Mary mentally transport herself to her last birthday party, which had been a very pleasant experience for her. The treatment planned for the visit was then accomplished by using local anaesthesia. At each subsequent visit, a previously spoken signal made her induction almost instantaneous (pp. 12–13).

Preparing the patient
Most patients, whether they be medical or dental, often have little idea of what is going to happen to them when they seek professional care. When medical patients consult a general practitioner or a hospital specialist, it is more than likely that they will not know what is the cause of their discomfort, its seriousness, or what procedures may be necessary to alleviate the problem. A medical illness is particularly anxiety-provoking if hospitalization is required since the disease could be life-threatening and almost certainly disruptive to the family concerned.

There is now an extensive literature which has explored the effects of preparing patients for such procedures as termination of pregnancy, gastrointestinal endoscopy, barium enemas, intrauterine device insertion, cast removal and a variety of surgical procedures. In an early and influential study (Egbert et al., 1964), one group of patients were given only the basic information usually provided—the time and duration of the operation and that they would waken from the anaesthesia in a recovery room. A second group of patients was given this basic preparation plus some additional information, including:

1. A description of the postoperative pain, including where it would be localized, how much could be expected and how long it would continue.
2. Reassurance that postoperative pain was normal and could be expected.
3. Advice on how to relax abdominal muscles and how to move without tensing them (all patients had abdominal operations).
4. Assurance that they would be given pain-killing medication should they require it.

This extra preparation thus provided more accurate expectations about what was to come and ways of coping. The results were quite striking. The fully prepared group required only half as much morphine during the first 5 postoperative days and had an average 2.7 fewer days of hospitalization.

There have been several explanations for such results. Janis (1971) argued that patients who were informed about their operations were able to engage in what he called 'the work of worrying', a kind of inner preparation for the stress to come. Patients could plan their coping methods and rehearse them mentally if they knew what to expect. This explanation fits well with a study mentioned in Chapter 4, where the recovery of children who were given 1 week's notice of an extraction was quicker than the recovery of children who were told only on the day of the extraction (Baldwin and Barnes, 1966). Those given prior notice expressed a wish 'to think about it' and 'get ready for it'. Another explanation involves the reduction of anxiety. A patient who is not informed about how he or she will be treated and feel afterwards has to contend with much uncertainty, and this may increase the amount of pain experienced. A third explanation involves control: a patient who can predict what is going to happen has more opportunity to exert control than someone who has little idea about the treatment.

Whichever of these (related) explanations finds the most favour, the evidence supports the idea that most patients can be helped with their pain by informing them about what they can expect (Reading, 1979). There are still many unanswered questions (such as the effects of using the word 'pain' to describe what they will feel), but the general direction of findings is reasonably clear. Unfortunately, there are very few examples of this kind of research applied to dental patients. One example has been given by Wardle (1982). Her study was mentioned earlier in the chapter under 'Enhancing control' and involved assessing the usefulness of a stop signal for relieving pain. In another condition of the same experiment, she asked the dentists to give a running commentary on their work as they performed it: what they were doing, when some discomfort could be expected and when their work would be definitely pain-free. When the amount of pain felt by this group of patients was compared with those given routine care, 50% of the latter group reported some pain, but only 22% of those who were informed as to what to expect.

Summary

The amount of pain a person feels cannot be predicted from knowledge of the stimulus alone. Many other factors influence the experience of pain, including the meaning of the situation, personality variables and culture. There are indications that people learn to respond to some kinds of stimulation as though they are painful. This learning could take place through the observation of friends and relatives. Gate Theory has three implications:

1 that all pains have both psychogenic and somatogenic features;
2 that the experience of pain is partly dependent on previous learning;
3 that research on pain conducted in the laboratory may not apply to real-life situations.

These multiple influences on pain make measurement difficult. Physiological measures, such as the amount of perspiration and heart rate, provide one means of measurement. Self-reports can also be used. These include asking the patient to indicate the amount of pain felt on a 10-cm line, and the McGill Pain Questionnaire, where the patient is asked to choose adjectives which best describe the pain. Another approach is behavioural. Here, the amount of analgesic given by staff or requested by patients could be monitored.

According to Gate Theory, psychological techniques should be effective in relieving pain for dental patients. The sensory–discriminative component can be altered through relaxation. Distraction and giving the patient some control over the dentist's behaviour are effective in alleviating pain on the affective–emotional dimension. The cognitive–evaluative component is affected by expectations about pain, so that the use of the word 'pain' itself may not always be helpful. Hypnosis and providing patients with information about their treatment can also be effective. Whenever testing the effectiveness of a technique for alleviating pain it is important to include a placebo control group.

Practice implications

1 Pain, like anxiety, is a private experience. Although there are verbal and non-verbal correlates of discomfort, a dentist may not always have an accurate view of the degree of pain a patient is feeling.
2 There are a number of straightforward psychological techniques which dentists can use to decrease discomfort. The patient can be involved in making a choice between methods.

Suggested reading

Melzack and Wall's *The Challenge of Pain* (Harmondsworth, Penguin, 1982) provides an interesting introduction to the neurological aspects of pain. For a more psychologically based view, Sternbach R.A. (ed.) *The Psychology of Pain*, (New York, Raven Press, 1978) is recommended.

References

Baldwin D. C., Barnes M. L. (1966) The psychological value of a presurgical waiting period in the preparation of children for dental extraction. *Trans. Eur. Orthodont., pp. Soc.* 297–308.
Beecher H. K. (1946) Pain in men wounded in battle. *Ann. Surg.* **128,** 96–105.
Bergner M., Bobbitt R. (1981) The Sickness Impact Profile: development and final revision of a health status measure. *Med. Care* **19,** 787–805.
Bond, M. R. (1979) *Pain*. Edinburgh: Churchill Livingstone.
Bond M. R. (1980) Personality and pain. In *Persistent Pain, Vol. 2* (Lipton S., ed.). London: Academic Press.
Bond M. R., Pilowski I. (1966) Subjective assessment of pain and its relationship to the administration of analgesics in patients with advanced cancer. *J. Psychosom. Res.* **10,** 203–8.

Burstein A., Burstein M. (1979) Injection pain: memory, expectation and experienced pain. *N.Y. J. Dent.* **49**, 183–5.
Coe W. C. (1980) Expectations, hypnosis and suggestion in behaviour change. In *Helping People Change* (Kanier F. H., Goldstein A. P., eds). Oxford: Pergamon.
Dangott L., Thornton B. C., Page P. (1978) Communication and pain. *J. Commun.* **28**, 30–5.
Dubuisson D., Melzack R. (1976) Classification of clinical pain description by multiple group discrimination analysis. *Exp. Neurol.* **51**, 480–7.
Dworkin S. F., Chen A. C. H. (1982) Pain in clinical and laboratory contexts. *J. Dent. Res.* **61**, 772–4.
Dworkin S. F., Ference T. P., Giddon D. B. (1978) *Behavioral Science and Dental Practice.* St Louis, Mosby.
Egbert L. D., Battit E. W., Welch C. E. et al. (1964) Reduction of post-operative pain by encouragement and instruction of patients. *N. Engl. J. Med.* **270**, 825–7.
Ekman P. (1973) *Darwin and Facial Expressions.* London: Academic Press.
Engstrom D. R. (1976) Hypnotic susceptibility, EEG alpha and self-regulation. In *Consciousness and Self-regulation* (Schwartz G. E., Shapiro D., eds). London: Plenum Press.
Eysenck H. (1967) *The Biological Basis of Personality.* Springfield, Illinois: Thomas.
Fier M. A. (1980) Hypnosis in dentistry: a case history. *Dent. Surv.* **56**, 12–13.
Fuller H. P., Menke R. A., Meyers W. J. (1979) Perception of pain to three different intra-oral penetrations of needles. *J. Am. Dent. Assoc.* **99**, 822–4.
Gardner W. J., Licklinder J. C. R. (1959) Auditory analgesia in dental operations. *J. Am. Dent. Assoc.* **59**, 1144–9.
Grushka M., Sessle B.J. (1984) Applicability of the McGill Pain Questionnaire to the differentiation of 'toothache' pain. *Pain* **19**, 49–57.
Hilgard E. R. (1975) The alleviation of pain by hypnosis. *Pain* **1**, 213–31.
Horan J. J., Layng F. C., Pursell C. H. (1976) Preliminary study of 'in vivo' emotive imagery on dental discomfort. *Percept. Mot. Skills* **42**, 105–6.
Houde R. W., Wallerstein S. L., Rogers M. (1960) Clinical pharmacology of analgesics. *Clin. Pharmacol. Ther.* **1**, 163–71.
Jan H. (1964) General semantic orientation in dentist–patient relations. *J. Am. Dent. Assoc.* **68**, 424–9.
Janis I. L. (1971) *Stress and Frustration.* New York: Harcourt Brace Jovanovich.
Kent G. (1986) Hypnosis in dentistry *Br. J. Exp. Clin. Hyp.* **3**, 103–112.
Kleck R. E., Vaughan R. C., Cartwright-Smith J. et al. (1976) Effects of being observed on expressive, subjective and physiological responses to painful stimuli. *J. Pers. Soc. Psychol.* **34**, 1211–18.
Klepac R. K., Dowling J., Hauge G. et al. (1980a) Reports of pain after dental treatment, electrical tooth pulp stimulation and cutaneous shock. *J. Am. Dent. Assoc.* **100**, 692–5.
Klepac R. K., McDonald M., Hauge G. et al. (1980b) Reactions to pain among subjects high and low in dental fear. *J. Behav. Med.* **3**, 373–84.
Klepac R. K., Dowling J., Hauge G. (1982) Characteristics of clients seeking therapy for the reduction of dental avoidance: reactions to pain. *J. Behav. Ther. Exp. Psychiatry* **13**, 293–300.
Kosambi D. D. (1967) Living prehistory in India. *Sci. Am.* **216**, 105–14.
Langer E., Janis I., Wolper J. (1975) Reduction of psychological stress in surgical patients. *J. Exp. Soc. Psychol.* **11**, 155–65.
Lanzetta J. T., Cartwright-Smith J., Kleck R. E. (1976) Effects of non-verbal dissimulation on emotional experience and autonomic arousal. *J. Pers. Soc. Psychol.* **33**, 354–70.
Lautch H. (1971) Dental phobia. *Br. J. Psychiatry* **119**, 151–8.
Leiderman P. H., Shapiro D. (1965) *Psychobiological Approaches to Social Behaviour.* London: Tavistock Publications.
Levine J.D., Gordon J., Fields H. (1978) The mechanism of placebo analgesia. *Lancet* **2**, 654–7.
Melzack R. (1975) The McGill Pain Questionnaire: major properties and scoring methods. *Pain* **1**, 279–99.

Melzack R., Loeser J. D. (1978) Phantom body pain in paraplegics: evidence for a central 'pattern generating mechanism' for pain. *Pain* **4**, 195–210.
Melzack R., Wall P. (1982) *The Challenge of Pain.* Harmondsworth: Penguin.
Melzack R., Taenzer P., Feldman P. et al. (1981) Labour is still painful after childbirth training. *Can. Med. Assoc. J.* **125**, 357–63.
Melzack R., Weisz A. Z., Sprague L. T. (1963) Strategies for controlling pain: contributions of auditory stimulation and suggestion. *Exp. Neurol.* **8**, 239–47.
Neiberger E. J. (1978) Child response to suggestion. *J. Dent. Child.* **45**, 396–402.
Parbrook G. D., Steel D. F., Dalrymple D. G. (1973) Factors predisposing to postoperative pain and pulmonary complications. *Br. J. Anaesth.* **45**, 21–33.
Pearce S., Erskine A. (1989) Chronic pain. In *The Practice of Behavioural Medicine* (Pearce S., Wardle J., eds). Oxford: British Psychological Society.
Phillips H. (1989) Thoughts provoked by pain. *Behav. Res. Ther.* **27**, 469–73.
Reading A. E. (1979) The short-term effects of psychological preparation for surgery. *Soc. Sci. Med.* **13A**, 641–54.
Reading A. E. (1980) A comparison of pain rating scales. *J. Psychosom. Res.* **24**, 119–24.
Scott P. J., Huskisson E. C. (1976) Graphic representation of pain. *Pain* **2**, 175–84.
Shapiro A. K., Morris L. A. (1978) The placebo effect in medical and psychological therapies. In *Handbook of Psychotherapy and Behaviour Change,* 2nd edn (Garfield S., Bergin A. E., eds). Chichester: Wiley.
Simmel M. L. (1962) The reality of phantom sensations. *Social Res.* **29**, 337–56.
Smith S.R. (1987) Hypnosis in general dental practice. In *The 1987 Dental Annual* (Derrick D., ed.). Bristol: Wright.
Thompson S. C. (1981) Will it hurt less if I can control it? A complex answer to a simple question. *Psychol. Bull.* **90**, 89–101.
Thrash W. J., Marr J. N., Boone S. E. (1982a) Continuous self-monitoring of discomfort in the dental chair and feedback to the dentist. *J. Behav. Assess.* **4**, 273–84.
Thrash W. J., Marr J. H., Box T. G. (1982b) Effects of continuous patient information in the dental environment. *J. Dent. Res.* **61**, 1063–5.
Van Buren J., Kleinknecht R. A. (1979) An evaluation of the McGill Pain Questionnaire for use in dental pain. *Pain* **6**, 23–33.
Wardle J. (1982) *Management of Dental Pain.* Paper presented at the British Psychological Society Annual Conference, York, 1982.
Weitzenhoffer A. M., Hilgard E. R. (1959) *Stanford Hypnotic Susceptibility Scale.* Palo Alto: Consulting Psychologists Press.
Zola J. K. (1966) Culture and symptoms: an analysis of patients' presenting complaints. *Am. Sociol. Rev.* **31**, 615–30.

Chapter 6

Special groups

The purpose of this chapter is to consider some groups of patients who have particular dental and personal needs. In a very real sense, of course, each patient is 'special' with his or her unique problems, but it does seem useful to consider some patients as having certain problems in common. Many groups could be discussed. Patients with medical problems such as cardiac, haemophilia, asthma and central nervous system conditions present psychological as well as physiological difficulties for the dentist (Hall, 1979; Swallow and Swallow, 1980). In addition, patients who are human immunodeficiency virus antibody-positive will present ethical and confidentiality problems (Glick, 1990). For patients with certain medical problems, the timing of appointments could be very important. Patients with arthritis or those who have had a colostomy might require an afternoon appointment, while someone with a kidney dysfunction could prefer a morning appointment (Ettinger et al., 1979). Patients who are immunocompromised (such as children on chemotherapy) might need appointments when the waiting room is empty to reduce the risk of picking up an infection. A child who is chronically ill and requires constant medication is under a greater risk of caries development if the medical practitioner does not prescribe sugar-free medication. A physical handicap may reduce the ability to keep teeth clean: an electric toothbrush provides a partial solution to such a problem but perhaps the most important contribution a dentist can make in such instances is preventive advice, stressing the importance of reducing sugar in the diet and encouraging the use of fluoride supplements.

In discussing special groups of patients, it is useful to remember the distinction between impairment, disability and handicap mentioned in Chapter 1. The term 'impairment' is used to refer to any psychological, physiological or anatomical loss or abnormality of structure or function. A 'disability' refers to the type of limitation imposed by the impairment, while the term 'handicap' refers to the difficulty a person has in fulfilling his or her roles within a family or society. Four groups of patients with varying types of impairment, disability and handicap are considered in this chapter: orthodontic patients, patients with temporomandibular joint (TMJ) and mandibular pain dysfunction (MPD) difficulties, elderly people, and people with a mental handicap.

Orthodontics

Research on psychological aspects of orthodontic treatment has been conducted in three main areas. One involves a consideration of the factors which influence the decision to seek treatment. As discussed in Chapter 1, this is often made by parents or a dentist rather than by patients themselves. Two other areas concern the lack of co-operation sometimes shown by children and adolescents and the psychological and social effects of treatment.

Co-operation with treatment

It seems that most orthodontists have difficulty with some of their patients due to a lack of co-operation, mainly with a refusal to wear headgear. Dental indices of the severity of malocclusion are not related to co-operation (McDonald, 1973), but the *patient's* perception of severity does show a relationship. Co-operative patients are more likely to be sensitive to their facial appearance and to be co-operative in other spheres, such as school (Clemmer and Hayes, 1979). El-Mangoury (1981) reports an interesting study on patients with class II malocclusions. Co-operation was measured by the amount of headgear wear, appliance maintenance, frequency of broken appointments and oral hygiene. Personality measures were also taken. An especially relevant personality characteristic was the patient's concern and desire for close personal relationships—called affiliation motivation—which was the best predictor of co-operation. Those patients for whom relationships were very important were most likely to be co-operative. This could reflect a recognition of the role of appearance in relationships or it could reflect a more general tendency to try and get along with everyone, including the dentist.

One factor which may be very important for co-operation relates to the decision to seek treatment initially. Often a parent or a dentist initiates the decision to have orthodontic care, yet it is the child who has to bear the consequences. Perhaps patients who receive treatment because their patents or dentist believe it is important but who do not share this belief tend to be unco-operative. In other areas of health care patients who seek help because of their own wishes are often more co-operative than those who are sent by other members of the family. Co-operation might be increased by discussing such issues with the patient at the beginning of treatment.

Effects of treatment

This aspect of orthodontic care has received increasing examination in recent years. There is much evidence that an individual's physical attractiveness has a significant effect on how he or she is perceived by others. A method which is frequently used in psychology experiments in this area is to present photographs to people and ask questions concerning expectations about those portrayed. Some photographs would show physically attractive individuals while others depict less attractive people. Expectations about personality (e.g. would this person be warm and friendly or cold and aggressive?) could be measured. The question is whether appearance affects expectations. In one of the more consistently replicated findings in psychology, attractive people are seen more positively than unattractive ones.

Shaw (1981) hypothesized that children with normal dental appearance would be judged as better looking and more socially attractive than those with dental anomalies. He altered photographs to show normal incisors; prominent incisors; a missing upper left lateral incisor; severely crowded incisors, and a unilateral cleft palate. Children shown these photographs were asked questions like: 'If this boy (girl) was coming to your class, do you think you would like him (her) as a friend?', and adults were asked questions like 'Do you think this boy (girl) would attract friends easily?' As predicted, children with normal incisors were rated as being more socially attractive, by both children and adults, than those shown in other photographs.

A related question is whether orthodontic treatment can affect attractiveness as measured in this way. Korabik (1981) was able to show that it does by asking people to view photographs of the same patients taken before or after treatment: the pretreatment photographs were rated as being significantly less attractive than the post-treatment ones. In another study using the same photographs patients were rated as being more intelligent and well adjusted after treatment. In both these experiments the photos portrayed differences in facial structure rather than dentition since the mouths were closed and the configuration of the teeth was not apparent.

Although this type of research provides consistent support for a link between orthodontic treatment, perceived attractiveness and liking, the 'real' significance of the results is open to question. Most of the studies are rather artificial, relying on photographs, and usually no additional information about the individuals is provided. In real life, of course, the situation is different. Dentition is only one source of information about someone. As we get to know a person better any malocclusion becomes insignificant, and there are some studies (e.g. Shaw and Humphreys, 1982) which indicate that when further information about patients shown on photographs is given the dentition becomes relatively insignificant. On the other hand, people can be very self-conscious about their teeth, so that orthodontic care may increase self-confidence even if it has little effect on others' perceptions.

Self-confidence
Although one would expect that self-confidence and self-esteem would rise after treatment, this has not been shown. Klima et al. (1979) examined satisfaction with body image and self-concept in three groups of children. One group was about to complete their orthodontic treatment, a second group consisted of new patients, and the third group was a control, made up of children not requiring assistance. The prediction that the second group would be the most dissatisfied with their appearance and have the most negative self-concept was not supported: there were no differences between the groups on the measures taken.

Since one of the main justifications for orthodontic treatment is that psychological benefits will accrue, the lack of support found in Klima et al.'s and other studies (e.g. Rutzen, 1973) has led to some questioning of the underlying assumption that people are handicapped by malocclusion. Only one study seems to have addressed this specifically: Kenealy et al. (1989) took a wide range of measures of 1018 children between 11 and 12 years of age. The measures included dentists' ratings of malocclusion, teachers' ratings of attractiveness, the children's own self-ratings of attractiveness and children's self-esteem. None of these measures correlated with each other particularly well. For example, the dentists' ratings of malocclusion correlated only 0.009 with children's self-ratings of attractiveness and 0.032 with their self-esteem. Although it can be argued that malocclusion was relatively unimportant for these children because they had not yet reached adolescence, when self-consciousness typically increases, this study provided no evidence that, overall, children suffer from having malocclusion. Research which distinguishes between malocclusion (the impairment), the limitations it imposes (the disability) and its social effects (the handicap) may be more successful in showing an effect for orthodontic care. Since these children are to be followed up over a number of years, a later study may provide more information.

Temporomandibular joint disorders

One problem in discussing the psychological aspects of TMJ disorders and the chronic pain sometimes associated with them is that of definition. Different investigators have taken various symptoms as indicators of TMJ problems, making it difficult to compare the results of different studies. Generally speaking, though, there is some agreement that a patient should show at least one of the following three symptoms before TMJ disorders (including MPD syndrome) is diagnosed:

1 pain and tenderness in the region of the muscles of mastication and temporomandibular joints;
2 limitations of mandibular movement;
3 sounds during condylar movement.

Aetiology

The aetiology of TMJ disorders has proven to be complex. Structural factors seem to be important for some patients but they do not provide a full explanation of TMJ problems, since no anatomical abnormalities can be found in many cases by methods available in the past.

Personality
This has led to an examination of personality and other psychological differences between TMJ and other dental patients. Many dentists have noted that people presenting with TMJ disorders are somehow 'psychologically different'. A wide variety of personality tests and psychiatric interviews have been used in an attempt to confirm this subjective impression and Rugh and Solberg (1976) provide a review of these studies.

They could find little consistency between results. TMJ patients have been found to be 'dependent, narcissistic, obsessive, sadistic, rigid, domineering, managerial, autocratic, perfectionistic, hypernormal, responsible, overgenerous, aggressive, proper, imaginative, neurotic, emotionally unstable, insecure, hypochondriacal and depressed' (p. 9). It is difficult to form a coherent picture from such a varied and sometimes contradictory profile. Perhaps the most important similarity between these adjectives is that most have very negative connotations, perhaps a reflection of the frustration that dentists can sometimes feel when trying to help this group of patients.

It is important to remember two problems with such studies. One problem is that most studies have examined patients who have sought help for their difficulties. As pointed out in Chapter 1, the prevalence of TMJ problems in the general population is quite high: perhaps researchers are discovering the types of people who seek help for their difficulties, rather than discovering anything about the aetiology of the condition itself. A second problem is that, even when a non-patient population is examined (Laan et al., 1987), assessments of personality have been made *after* the onset of the difficulties. Although there is a high rate of psychiatric problems in this group (Hughes et al., 1989), it is not possible to say that any personality characteristic is responsible for the condition. In Chapter 5 it was pointed out that chronic pain has a number of negative psychological effects, including depression, so it is equally likely that any differences which are found between TMJ and other patients could be due to the condition, rather than being responsible for it.

Stress

A much more fruitful approach has involved the possibility that TMJ problems are stress-related. The term 'stress' has been used in two ways. Sometimes it has been used to refer to the reaction of the organism, and sometimes to the external events which lead to some internal reaction. There is a substantial literature on how stressful experiences (ranging from such severe events as a death in the family or loss of employment to more everyday events such as taking an examination or receiving a parking ticket) can increase the likelihood that a person will consult a doctor or dentist. But it is not always clear whether a stressful event makes it more likely that a person will actually contract a disease or whether an event makes a person less able to cope with an already-present disability. For example, a person may manage to cope with a chronic pain until a stressful event occurs, such as a death in the family. This event would require the use of many psychological resources, making it more difficult to cope with the pain. Recently however there has been increasing evidence that the actual disease process is affected. It seems that stress can affect the immune system: several studies have shown that immunodeficiency can occur after the death of a close relative (for example, Kent and Dalgleish, 1986).

The experience of stress has also been implicated with the onset and maintenance of TMJ problems. First, there is evidence that stressful events lead to muscle tension. Both laboratory (Thomas et al., 1973) and naturalistic studies have found that TMJ patients often tense their jaw muscles when under stress. Rugh (1977) asked patients to wear a portable electromyogram recorder (a device to measure muscle activity) on their jaw muscles. The recorder would emit a warning tone whenever the electromyogram level was high, thus providing the patients with information about when they clenched their teeth. Most patients reported that the tone would sound during situations which they found stressful or emotionally arousing, such as driving, seeing their employers, or when the children came home from school. The incidence of bruxism in TMJ patients provides further evidence of a link with stress. It seems that TMJ patients are likely to react to stress by tooth-clenching: Grieder et al. (1971) found that 97 of 100 patients showed indications of bruxism, while in Ramfjord's (1961) sample of 37 patients all had clinical signs of tooth-grinding.

It now seems likely that a TMJ problem in a particular patient is often due to some combination of structural and stress-related factors. Not all patients clench their teeth under stress, nor does everyone with high electromyogram levels have TMJ disorders. But a combination of these two factors increases the likelihood of TMJ problems.

Treatment

These studies on aetiology provide some useful pointers towards effective therapy. Pharmacological approaches, stress management and counselling are three types of treatment.

Antidepressants
Tricyclic antidepressants, particularly amitriptyline, have been used with success in the treatment of pain associated with TMJ problems. They seem to have the ability to relieve pain independent of their antidepressant effect (Kriesberg, 1988). However there are three important arguments against relying wholly on pharmacological agents. First, they treat only the symptom and not the cause of the difficulty. Although medication may give palliative relief, the patient may become dependent on continuing dosages unless further steps are taken (Feinmann, 1989). Second, they can have toxic side-effects and so close monitoring is required. Third, when a drug is prescribed for the control of a personal or interpersonal problem, there is the implication that the problem is biological in origin and the patients' responsibility to examine and alter the way they react is reduced.

Stress management
The association between stress, muscle tension and symptoms suggests that many patients could be helped if they learnt to identify their sources of stress and react to them differently. Gessell and Alderman (1971) used the muscle relaxation techniques discussed in Chapter 4 and found them effective for most patients, while Cohen and Hillis (1979) found that hypnosis could be beneficial. In Rugh's (1977) study mentioned above, where patients were asked to wear an electromyogram monitor during the day, patients became aware of how often and in

which situations their jaw muscles were tensed. Rugh and his patients explored new ways of responding to these situations. Ten of the 15 patients showed significant clinical improvement in their symptoms after this intervention.

Charting can be accomplished even without the use of such equipment. For at least some patients, there is a fairly close relationship between pain and clenching, so that they could be asked to keep a record of the amount of pain they feel throughout the day and to note the circumstances which precede this pain. The chart shown in Table 6.1 could be used in this way. At the end of each hour the patient places a cross on the 100-mm line indicating the severity of pain and noting the events which had occurred. Then it is easy to take a ruler and measure the distance from one end to give a score from 0 to 100. This idea of charting tension and situations is mentioned again in the next chapter, where it is discussed in relation to dentists' own stress.

Table 6.1 A chart which could be used for monitoring the severity of pain and the circumstances in which it occurs. The patient places a cross on the 100 mm line indicating the severity of pain and makes a note of any important events in the past hour

Time	Day _____ Amount of pain		Circumstances
9.00	None	(100 mm)	Severe
10.00	None		Severe
11.00	None		Severe

Counselling

A third approach to alleviating TMJ difficulties is counselling. While the results of studies on stress management are very encouraging, the method does not work for everyone. It may be that patients who do not improve with this method are reluctant to consider the possibility that their TMJ problems may be psychologically based. Of the 5 treatment failures in the Gessell and Alderman (1971) study, 3 were under the care of a psychiatrist for depression and the other 2 were considered in need of psychiatric assistance. Counselling often focuses on interpersonal problems, because many of the stresses that people encounter involve conflicts with other people. This suggests that if patients can be helped to improve the quality of their relationships then the stressful nature of their lives may be reduced.

Pomp (1974) describes an effective course of help for 23 patients who did not respond to other types of treatment. During the first of 12 weekly sessions, patients were told about the relationship between emotional stress, muscular tension and jaw pain. They were assured that the pain was not imaginary and that their difficulties would be taken seriously. Counselling was suggested as a way of focusing on stress in their lives and the remaining sessions were devoted to this kind of discussion. Fifteen patients showed complete remission of symptoms, often quite quickly. Other somatic difficulties (e.g. headaches) also cleared up. Pomp considered those who did not improve or who dropped out before the end of the 12 sessions to have more severe emotional difficulties.

The elderly patient

Chronological age is a poor predictor of an individual's capabilities. The evidence that elderly people are less able than the young comes mainly from studies in which young and old are compared on cognitive or physiological measures. Elderly people tend to do less well on intelligence tests of certain kinds, on reaction time tests, where a light is flashed or a buzzer sounded and the task is to press a button as quickly as possible, on visual adaptation, hearing, and so on. However such results are based on *group* scores: there are many elderly people who perform better on such tests than many young people. For example, age-related differences in physiological capabilities have been found between healthy men over the age of 65 and athletic males aged 19–22, but little difference between these elderly people and non-athletic young men. Furthermore, older people can often perform as well as young people if they are given some additional practice. Thus it is important to make a distinction between those changes which occur concurrently with ageing (e.g. a decline in oral health) but are not due to the ageing process itself (Gilbert, 1989). It is also important to realize that only a minority of elderly people suffer from such problems as hearing loss, senility or deterioration of vision. Surveys have shown that the facts do not support the stereotype.

The view one holds of elderly people can have important effects on how they are treated. On the one hand, as discussed in Chapter 1, elderly people have the lowest utilization rate of all adults. This seems to be due in part to a belief held by many older people that they do not merit careful and attentive treatment. In our culture old age is seen as a negative attribute and being seen as old and useless can affect feelings of personal worth and self-esteem. Symptoms may be interpreted as a natural part of the ageing process, rather than a result of some disease process, so that care is not sought.

Views of elderly people may also affect the care given by professionals. If ageing is seen purely as a process of deterioration, then older people might be given a lower priority for scarce resources. Ettinger (1984) points out several ways in which preconceived notions about elderly people can affect care. For example, a clinician who realizes the hypothesis that salivary function declines with age has not been supported by research will be less likely to attribute a complaint of a dry mouth to old age and will consider a pathological process instead. A dentist may also be less likely to decline to give periodontal care to an 80-year-old if he or she realizes that the expected life span is another 8 years.

Edentulousness

As discussed in Chapter 1, edentulousness is increasingly becoming a condition found mainly in the elderly. This is due in part to changes in the dental profession's approach to care and in part to the lessening need for extractions due to caries. Some of the factors which relate to patients' acceptance of dentures were outlined in Chapter 1, and further studies which indicate that the dentist's approach is important are discussed in the next chapter.

Some mention here should be made of patients' reactions to edentulousness. Many people find the prospect of having their teeth removed a disturbing one. Friedman et al. (1987, 1988) discuss how tooth loss can represent a type of disfigurement that has implications for body image and self-esteem. Such a negative reaction may be more likely if the patient is already coping with other stressful life events, if tooth loss is seen as a sign of irrevocable loss of youth and function, or if there are already-existing problems with self-image. When wearing dentures many patients become very self-conscious and reticent in social situations. They may refuse invitations to dinner, avoid certain foods and become embarrassed if the topic is raised. Of central importance is the feeling that the appliance is a foreign object in the mouth. As one of Friedman et al.'s (1988) patients put it 'the denture fits, I am not suffering any physical pain but part of me is gone. These are not mine, they are a dead part of myself' (p. 88). A major advance in recent years is the development of osseointegrated implants, which appear to restore patients' functional abilities as well as reduce distress because they are integrated psychologically as well as anatomically (Blomberg and Linquist, 1983).

Patients with handicaps

There are many negative stereotypes in our society of people who behave 'differently' or look unusual. Those with a physical handicap or who are psychiatrically disabled are often stigmatized and avoided (Thomas, 1978; Jones et al., 1984). This can have several effects on the individual, including low self-esteem and a painful loneliness. Handicaps usually affect the functioning of families as well. The presence of a severe handicap in a newborn child can be devastating for parents and they may require considerable support.

Mental handicap

The presence of a mental handicap can be established through the use of IQ tests which are designed to measure an individual's capacity for learning, but in practice it is the ability to function in society which is of central importance. A person may have a low IQ score but be able to lead a reasonably independent life given adequate support. It is also important to point out that everyone requires support from others in order to function, so that handicap is a matter of degree rather than of kind. There is a wide range of ability in people with mental handicaps, from those who have difficulty with basic skills such as feeding and toileting to those who can lead an independent life. While the behaviour of some people with a mental handicap can be erratic and seemingly unpredictable, most do not show such disturbances.

Severe deficits can mean that people with a mental handicap have some problems not shared by other groups of dental patients. Toothbrushing is a very complex cognitive and motor task which may be beyond their capabilities. A companion may be needed to guide them to a dentist, to brush their teeth and to monitor their diet. Preventive dental care is especially important, particularly if the patient will not be able to wear dentures because of epileptic fits. Many of the principles outlined in Chapters 2 and 4 for encouraging oral health behaviours (Albino et al., 1979) and reducing disruptive behaviour (Dicks, 1974; Bloxham and Swallow, 1975) have been used with success. Regular inspections are vital since the most severely handicapped individuals will not be able to communicate directly that they have a toothache.

Until recently, people requiring residential care were housed in large hospitals, but over the past decades there have been attempts to provide an environment which is as similar as possible to that of non-handicapped people. Instead of large hospitals, smaller community-based hostels are being built, and in some areas houses have been converted to allow residents to be as fully integrated with the community as their disabilities allow. This change in policy has been due in part to the recognition that living in large institutions can lead to a deterioration of abilities and in part to the recognition that it is unethical to limit a person's autonomy unnecessarily.

There has been a corresponding move to encourage general dental practitioners to treat patients with a mental handicap in their offices. To this end, a few dental schools include in their curricula visits to local hostels and hospitals in order to acquaint students with the problems of treating this group of patients and to dispel any myths which might discourage the students from treating them in the future. At one dental school, for instance, two-thirds of the students had reservations about treating patients with a mental handicap, partly because they 'didn't know what to expect, had preconceived ideas about the patients being uncommunicative and disruptive, and were afraid that they could not handle the work emotionally or physically' (Block and Walken, 1980, p. 161). After having visited a local hospital and given restorations with the help of a well trained dental auxiliary, 95% said that they would now be willing to treat these patients in their private practice. As one student put it, 'I became aware that unless the patients had some complicated medical problems, they are no more difficult to treat than normal patients'. The expectation that people with a mental handicap are difficult to treat has been examined further by Melville et al. (1981). They set up a mobile service for handicapped children: only 8.5% of the children could not be treated with this facility and were referred to the local dental hospital for treatment.

Davies et al. (1988) interviewed parents and dentists about their views on dental treatment for mentally handicapped adults. Many of the parents believed that regular attendance was important for the maintenance of function (30%), clear speech (20%) and aesthetics (43%), but these aspects were less important for dentists, who emphasized the prevention of periodontal disease. Both dentists and patients believed that lack of experience with mentally handicapped people was an important problem, but for the dentists the most important problems concerned the time that the care of handicapped patients might involve, which could interfere with their efficiency. Davies et al. suggest that payment on a sessional basis could help to alleviate this difficulty

The dentally handicapped patient
Brown (1980) has introduced the idea of the 'dentally handicapped' patient. For any one of several reasons—such as mental handicap, excessive fear of dentistry, haemophilia, heart disease—a patient may be unable to receive routine dental care. In such instances preventive care is crucial. In his study of 53 dentally handicapped children, parents co-operated in controlling diet and using electric toothbrushes and fluoride tablets. Over the course of the study there was a marked decrease in carious lesions and a corresponding increase in oral health for these children. Moreover, this programme was shown to have cost benefits, with the preventive care costing considerably less than the expected number of restorations. The involvement of parents in such a programme is clearly essential, particularly where diet is concerned.

Summary

It is often inappropriate to make generalizations about patients who share a particular condition since two people may have the same objective impairment but be disabled or handicapped in different ways. How an individual reacts and attends to an impairment are important psychological factors during treatment. Although studies have indicated that the social and psychological effects of orthodontic work seem to be minimal for many people, it is likely that patients who are very self-conscious of the appearance of their teeth will benefit. Others may not. TMJ disorders appear to result from a combination of factors such as morphology, levels of stress and the individual's ways of coping with stress. Some elderly people seem to take on the cultural view that they are less worthwhile than the young and do not want to 'bother' the dentist despite the presence of severe symptoms. People with a mental handicap are sometimes unable to seek treatment themselves, relying on the vigilance of others.

Practice implications

1 In orthodontic care it is important to assess the patient's view of the need for treatment and the psychological costs of wearing an appliance.
2 TMJ patients can be helped by reviewing their life stresses and offering more adaptive ways of coping.
3 Elderly patients may be reluctant to seek care. On the other hand it is important not to put pressure on them to undergo treatment when they have adapted to their oral state.

4 There are many negative but unfounded stereotypes about people with a mental handicap. Most such people can be treated in private practice, but some will require additional teaching when it comes to learning new skills.

Suggested reading

The Dental Clinics of North America series (London: Saunders) provide useful sources of information on specific topics. Terezhalmy G.T. and Saunders M. (1989) *Geriatric Dentistry* and Schlossberg A. (1990) *Controversies in Dentistry* cover some of the topics raised in this chapter.

References

Albino J.E., Schwartz B., Goldberg H., Stern R. (1979) Results of an oral hygiene programme for severely retarded children. *J. Dent. Child.* **46**, 25–9.
Block M.J., Walken J. (1980) Effects of an extra-mural programme on student attitudes towards dental care for the mentally retarded. *J. Dent. Educ.* **44**, 158–61.
Blomberg S., Linquist L. (1983) Psychological reactions to edentulousness and treatment with jawbone-anchored bridges. *Acta Psychiatr. Scand.* **68**, 251–62.
Bloxham E., Swallow J. (1975) The dental treatment of institutionalised mentally handicapped people. *Br. Dent. J.* **139**, 145–6.
Brown J.P. (1980) The efficacy and economy of comprehensive dental care for handicapped children *Int. Dent. J.* **30**, 14–27.
Clemmer E.J., Hayes E. (1979) Patient co-operation in wearing orthodontic headgear. *Am. J. Orthodont.* **75**, 517–24.
Cohen E.S., Hillis R.E. (1979) The use of hypnosis in treating the temporomandibular joint pain dysfunction syndrome. *Oral Surg.* **48**, 193–7.
Davies K.W., Holloway P., Worthington H. (1988) Dental treatment for mentally handicapped adults in general practice. *Community Dent. Health* **5**, 381–7.
Dicks J.L. (1974) Effects of different communication techniques on the co-operation of the mentally retarded child during dental procedures. *J. Dent. Child.* **41**, 283–8.
El-Mangoury N.H. (1981) Orthodontic co-operation. *Am. J. Orthodont.* **80**, 604–22.
Ettinger R.L. (1984) Clinical decision making in the dental treatment of the elderly. *Gerodontology* **3**, 157–65.
Ettinger R.L., Beck J., Glenn R. (1979) Eliminating office architectural barriers to dental care of the elderly and handicapped. *J. Am. Dent. Assoc.* **98**, 398–401.
Feinmann C. (1989) Diagnosis and management of TMJ problems by the general dental practitioner. In *The 1989 Dental Annual* (Derrick D., ed.). London: Wright.
Friedman N., Landesman H., Wexler M. (1987) The influence of fear, anxiety and depression on the patient's adaptive responses to complete dentures. Part 1. *J. Prosthet. Dent.* **58**, 687–9.
Friedman N., Landesman H., Wexler M. (1988) The influences of fear, anxiety and depression on the patient's adaptive responses to complete dentures. Part ll. *J. Prosthet. Dent.* **59**, 45–8.
Gessell A.H., Alderman M. (1971) Management of myofascial pain dysfunction syndrome of the temporomandibular joint by tension control training. *Psychosomatics* **12**, 302–9.
Gilbert G.H. (1989) 'Ageism' in dental care delivery. *J. Am. Dent. Assoc.* **118**, 545–8.
Glick M. (1990) HIV testing: more questions than answers. In *Controversies in Dentistry. Dental Clinics of North America*. (Schlossberg A., ed.) London: Saunders.
Grieder A., Vinton P., Cinotti W., Kangur T. (1971) An evaluation of ultrasonic therapy for temporomandibular joint dysfunction. *Oral Surg.* **31**, 25–31.

Hall R.K. (1979) Dental management of the chronically ill child. *Aust. Dent. J.* **24**, 334–41.

Hughes A.M., Hunter S., Still D., Lamey P. (1989) Psychiatric disorders in a dental clinic. *Br. Dent. J.* **166**, 16–19.

Jones E.E., Farina A., Hastorf A. et al (1984) *Social Stigma*. New York: Freeman.

Kenealy P., Frude N and Shaw W. (1989) An evaluation of the psychological and social effects of malocclusion: some implications for dental policy making. *Soc. Sci. Med.* **28**, 583–91.

Kent G., Dalgleish M. (1986) *Psychology and Medical Care*. London: Bailliere Tindall.

Klima R.J., Witteman J., McIver J. (1979) Body image, self-concept and the orthodontic patient. *Am. J. Orthodont.* **75**, 507–16.

Korabik K. (1981) Changes in physical attractiveness and interpersonal attraction. *Basic Appl. Soc. Psychol.* **2**, 59–65.

Kriesberg M.K. (1988) Tricyclic antidepressants: analgesic effect and indications in orofacial pain. *J. Craniomandib. Disord. Facial Oral Pain* **2**, 171–7.

McDonald F.T. (1973) The effect of age on patient co-operation in orthodontic treatment. *Dent. Abstr.* **18**, 52.

Melville M.R.B., Pool D.M., Jaffe E.C., Gelbier S., Tulley W.J. (1981) A dental service for handicapped children. *Br. Dent. J.* **151**, 259–61.

Pomp A.M. (1974) Psychotherapy for the myofacial pain-dysfunction syndrome: a study of factors coinciding with symptom remission. *J. Am. Dent. Assoc.* **89**, 629–32.

Ramfjord S.P. (1961) Dysfunctional temporomandibular joint and muscle pain. *J. Prosthet. Dent.* **11**, 353.

Rugh J.D. (1977) A behavioural approach to diagnosis and treatment of functional and oral disorders: biofeedback and self-control techniques. In *Biofeedback in Dentistry: Research and Clinical Applications* (Rugh J.D., Perlis D., Disraeli R., eds). Phoenix: Semandotics.

Rugh J.D., Solberg W. (1976) Psychological implications in temporomandibular pain and dysfunction. *Oral Sci. Rev.* **7**, 3–30.

Rutzen S.R. (1973) The social importance of orthodontic rehabilitation: report of a five year follow-up study. *J. Health Soc. Behav.* **14**, 233–40.

Shaw W.C. (1981) The influence of children's dentofacial appearance on their social attractiveness as judged by peers and lay adults. *Am. J. Orthodont.* **79**, 399–415.

Shaw W.C., Humphreys S. (1982) Influence of children's dentofacial appearance in teacher expectations. *Community Dent. Oral. Epidemiol.* **10**, 313–19.

Swallow J.N., Swallow B. (1980) Dentistry for physically handicapped children in the International Year of the Child. *Int. Dent. J.* **30**, 1–5.

Thomas D. (1978) *The Social Psychology of Childhood Disability*. London: Methuen.

Thomas L.J., Tiber N., Schireson S. (1973) The effects of anxiety and frustration on muscular tension related to the temporomandibular joint syndrome. *Oral Surg.* **36**, 763–8.

van der Laan G. J., Duinkerke A., Lutejin F., van de Poel A. (1987) Role of psychologic and social variables in TMJ pain dysfunction syndrome (PDS) symptoms. *Community Dent. Oral Epidemiol.* **16**, 274–7.

Chapter 7

The dentist–patient relationship

Previous chapters in this book have concentrated almost exclusively on patients—the reasons why they do (or do not) visit a dentist regularly, ways that preventive care can be encouraged, and methods for alleviating their anxiety and pain. Yet it seems clear that the dentist's attitudes, personality and behaviour are also of importance for the understanding of dental care. Many instances of this have been given previously, but another example has been provided by Gryll and Katahn (1978). They were interested in the effects of dentists' behaviour on the effectiveness of a placebo pill which was said to relieve pain. All of the patients in their study were due to have an injection in preparation for an extraction. A measure of anxiety was administered and the patients were asked to rate their fear of the injection. The patients were then assigned to one of several conditions. For some patients, the dentist was instructed to be very warm and friendly and to engage them in open and reassuring conversation; for other patients the dentist was to be more neutral, with limited verbal exchanges. Another variable tested in the same study was the enthusiasm of the dentist. Some patients were told: 'This is a recently developed pill that I've found to be very effective in reducing tension, anxiety and sensitivity to pain. It cannot harm you in any way. The pill becomes effective almost immediately'. Others were told: 'This is a recently developed pill which reduces tension, anxiety and sensitivity to pain in some people. Other people receive no benefit from it at all. I personally have not found it to be very effective. It cannot harm you in any way. The pill becomes effective almost immediately if it is going to have an effect'. In order to control for any effects of simply giving a pill, a third condition was included where the placebo was given but no analgesic properties were mentioned. Here, the dentist said: 'This is a recently developed pill that reduces the amount of saliva in your mouth. It cannot harm you in any way. The pill becomes effective almost immediately'.

After hearing one of these messages, the patients' anxiety and fear of the injection were again measured. Their anxiety was found to be reduced by both messages, which indicated that the pill could be useful in relieving anxiety, but most by the enthusiastic one. Fear of the injection decreased for those given the enthusiastic message, but not the unenthusiastic one. These results were not due simply to giving the pill, since there was little effect from the saliva message.

Gryll and Katahn took one other interesting measure, the amount of pain felt by the patients during the injection. Directly after receiving the local anaesthetic, they were asked to rate the pain on a 1—5 scale. Both the type of message about the pill and the warmth of the dentist had significant effects. When the pill was enthusiastically promoted, the patients reported less pain, and when the dentist was warm and friendly, rather than neutral, the patients said they experienced less discomfort. Thus, the attitudes shown by the dentist moderated the unpleasant effects of the injection.

In such ways, a dentist's characteristics are important for the understanding of dental care. The aim of this chapter is to explore the relationship between dentist and patient, particularly the ways the *dentist's* behaviour, feelings and beliefs affect the relationship. Research on patients' perceptions of their dentists, communication skills and stress in dentistry illustrate the importance of self-awareness for practice.

Patients' perceptions of dentists

There are several ways to examine patients' views of dental practice. Patients' choice of dentist and their satisfaction with the care they receive are influenced by several factors. Both technical skill and the dentist's manner affect whether an individual chooses one dentist rather than another and whether the patient decides to stay with that practice.

Choosing a dental practice

This choice is rarely random. One survey of patients (Garfunkel, 1980) found that only 1% had made contact simply through a telephone book. All of the others had attempted to discover some information about possible practices. The most frequent source of information was friends and relatives who were asked for their recommendation. The results of another survey are shown in Table 7.1. Here, members of the general public were asked: 'What do you look for in choosing a dentist?'. The most frequently cited factor was: 'Dentist's manner—puts you at your ease', while only 25% mentioned 'Qualification and ability' (Bulman et al., 1968).

Table 7.1 Percentages of the general population who cited various reasons for choosing their dentist

Reason	Percentage of people mentioning reason
Dentist's manner—puts you at your ease	35
Dentist who doesn't hurt you	31
Recommendation	27
Qualification and ability	25
Other reasons	23
Doesn't look for anything	13
No waiting	12

Percentages total more than 100 since some people mentioned more than one reason.
After Bulman et al. (1968), with permission.

Another way of ascertaining which characteristics are most important for patients is to ask what would cause them to lose confidence in their dentist. In an American survey (Kreisberg and Treiman, 1962), the most frequently cited reason was 'Treatment poorly executed', followed by the dentist's manner: someone who was rough and apparently unconcerned about any pain would cause them to lose confidence. Only about half the sample said that dentists explained enough about treatment and prevention.

A third method is to ask patients what would constitute an 'ideal' dentist. McKeithen (1966) asked her sample to 'Try to think of the best dentist you can imagine. What would he be like?' The dentist's personality and attitudes towards the patient were mentioned by 59%. This included the dentist being pleasant, friendly and sociable as well as understanding and supportive. This was closely followed by professional ability, including skill and technical competence. Ability to reduce fear and pain was another important factor. An ideal dentist should be gentle, reassuring and explain procedures. Having a professional attitude was the next most frequently mentioned characteristic. The ideal dentist was said to inspire trust and be confident as well as being careful and conscientious. A final category included such factors as cleanliness, efficiency and providing dental education.

Priorities for patients

Yet another approach which has been used to assess patients' perceptions is to ask them to give priority to alternative characteristics of dentists. When this was done with patients in Norway (Skogedal and Heloe, 1979), 60% gave first priority to skill: 'The dentist is accurate and works safely, making you trust his/her professional skills'. Thirty-three per cent gave their first priority to 'The dentist is understanding and kind and the treatment is performed without pain'. For 26% it was the dentist who 'Takes his/her time to listen and to discuss dental health problems, and he/she explains how dental disease may be prevented'. The final possibility, efficiency ('The dentist works rapidly and efficiently and waiting time is at a minimum'), was given first priority by only 18%. (These percentages add up to more than 100% because some patients gave more than one answer.)

There are some interesting differences between various groups in the emphasis they place on these characteristics. Jenny et al. (1973) asked parents about their reasons for being satisfied with their child's dentist. Parents of high socioeconomic status were more likely to cite professional competence as a reason for satisfaction, whereas parents of low socioeconomic status were more likely to mention the positive relationship between their child and the dentist. Similar results were found in interviews with people from the general population (Van Groenestijn et al., 1980). When asked 'What characteristics do you think the ideal dentist should have? Could you note the three most important to you, in order of importance?', those from a high socioeconomic level cited professional skill, friendliness and providing information in that order, while those from a low socioeconomic level said reassurance and friendliness were most important, followed by professional skills. Thus, the characteristic which seems most important to patients varies somewhat depending on how the questions are phrased and which groups of people are interviewed, but there does appear to be some consistency. Generally, technical skills seem most important, but these are closely followed by interpersonal abilities.

Patients' judgements of technical skill

This raises a most interesting question—how patients judge their dentists' technical competence. Since there can be much disagreement between dentists as to what constitutes a good restoration (Ludwick et al., 1964), lay-people could be expected to be less able to make the judgement. When Jenny et al. (1973) asked parents if they felt their children's dentist was a good one, some said that they could not make this judgement easily. One parent responded 'Good question. Really don't know. Does anyone really?' Another said 'I am unable to judge. Frankly, unless fillings fall out or she [the child] has toothaches, I can't tell good work from bad'. Nevertheless, in this survey professional competence was cited by over half of the parents as a reason for their satisfaction with their children's dentist. A formal comparison between patients' and professional views of quality was made by Abrams et al. (1986). After patients were asked to judge the quality of the restorations they had received, the patients were examined by dentists in order to gain a professional view. An extremely low correlation (0.065) was found between these two viewpoints.

These studies suggest that patients may use other information in order to make a judgement about technical skill. Observations about the dentist's surgery, age and interactional style seem to influence this. Jackson (1978a) asked (non-dental) students to rate the skill and competence of several hypothetical dentists. The students were shown photographs of three surgeries. One was quite old, with a straightbacked chair, a spitoon and a belt-driven drill. Another was a contemporary set-up, from a university dental clinic, and the third was ultramodern, with an abundance of plants and wood furnishings. The students inferred that the dentist with an ultramodern surgery would be more trustworthy, more skillful and have more general competence than the other two. The students were also given some snippets of conversation between these hypothetical dentists and their patients. For example, to a patient's comment that 'I know that it would be good if I brushed after lunch at school, but I usually forget or I don't have time', one dentist remarked: 'Really, you should just make a point of doing it—it's just too important to forget'; another said 'Many people feel that way at first, but you really can form the habit if you persevere, believe me'; and a third said 'Sometimes it's hard to begin a new habit'. The first kind of response seemed to indicate more skill than the others for a dentist in his mid 30s and late 50s, but not for a newly qualified dentist. For a younger dentist, the second reply ('Many people feel that way at first') was seen to indicate most competence.

Patients' judgements about competence have aroused much interest in medical care. There, too, the technical and interpersonal abilities of doctors are often cited as important factors in patients' choices and satisfaction. Generally, a high correlation is found between their satisfaction with interpersonal aspects of care and their satisfaction with technical care. There is some evidence that medical patients use perceptions of doctors' caring and sympathy to make judgements about technical skill (Ben-Sira, 1982).

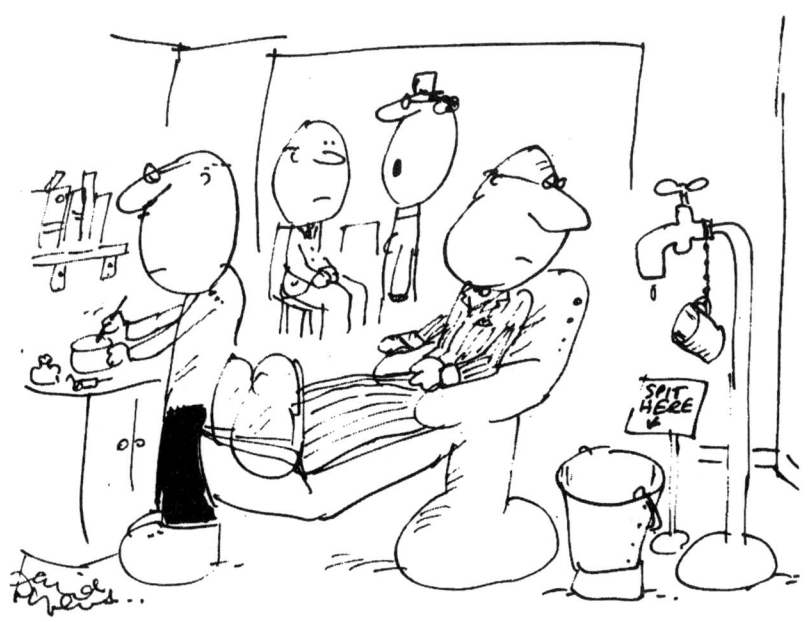

'He's inclined to be a shade mean where equipment is concerned...'
(Reproduced by permission of David Myers.)

Patient satisfaction

It is useful to make a distinction between cognitive and emotional satisfaction. The former relates to satisfaction with the information gathered about a problem: its cause, severity and prognosis. It is associated with the opportunity to ask questions and with the dentist's willingness to disclose information. Emotional satisfaction, on the other hand, refers to patients' feelings of trust towards the dentist. This is related to the chance to express worries and to the feeling of being understood (Stiles et al., 1979).

These two aspects of satisfaction are reflected in a study in which patients were asked about their experiences with dentists. In general, patients said that they liked the dentist to explain the treatment fully, to explain the use of equipment, and to be truthful. Conversely, dentists who started treatment without an explanation, who told them that a procedure that was actually painful would not hurt, and scolded them for poor oral hygiene were disliked (Rankin and Harris, 1985).

Satisfaction and attendance

Such research is of great interest, because satisfaction is related to compliance and appointment-keeping. In one survey (Kent, 1984), both dental patients and members of the general public were asked about their degree of satisfaction with dentists. As a measure of satisfaction, they were asked about the extent of their agreement or disagreement with a number of statements such as 'Most dentists take a real interest in their patients' and 'Dentists should be a little more friendly than they are' (Hengst and Roghmann, 1978). People who disagreed with statements like the first or agreed with statements like the second were less likely to attend a dentist for preventive check-ups and less likely to have attended within the previous 6 months.

In another study, patients' attendance at a student dental clinic was monitored. Patients who first agree to attend and then later drop out provide problems for both students and staff. Stacey et al. (1978) wanted to find out why some patients completed their treatment while others terminated prematurely. They posted questionnaires to both groups of patients asking them to indicate how they felt about several factors relating to their treatment. Then the authors tested for differences in how the two groups replied. The results are shown in Table 7.2. Generally speaking, the items can be subsumed under three factors, one having to do with treatment, another with ease of appointment keeping and a third with satisfaction with the interpersonal aspects of care.

This last aspect seems particularly important for irregular attenders. Further evidence for this comes from the study mentioned above where people were asked to give three characteristics of their ideal dentist in rank order (Van Groenestijn et al., 1980). Regular attenders tended to give first priority to skill, then friendliness and then reassurance. Irregular

Table 7.2 Factors which distinguished between patients who completed their treatment at a student dental clinic and those who terminated before the end of treatment

* Treatment wanted actually done
* Student's explanations understandable
  Tired of waiting for first appointment to be made
* Student concerned for my feelings
* Satisfaction with treatment
* Free time for appointments
* Helpfulness of clinic instructors
  Treatment took longer than expected
* Confidence in student's ability
  Inconvenient to pay for treatment with cash
  Trouble keeping appointments
  Difficulty in making appointments
  Wait for screening before first appointment
* Necessity of treatment planned
* Ability to co-operate in clinic
* Notice given before appointment
  Appointments hard to keep due to family situation

*Those factors on which patients who completed treatment scored more highly.
From Stacey et al. (1978), with permission.

attenders, on the other hand, ordered their priorities differently. For them, the order was friendliness, reassurance and then skill.

Dentists' perceptions of patients

Of course, there is the other side of the coin to consider—dentists' perceptions of their patients. Wills (1978) provides an interesting review of the literature concerning how members of the caring professions view their clients. He identified three dimensions which seemed to be important whatever the specialty. One dimension was manageability: the 'good patient' is one who follows instructions and is willing to assume the role of a patient. A second dimension was treatability. The 'good patient' demonstrates high motivation for treatment and although he or she might have some interesting problems these should not be too severe or difficult to treat. A third, attractiveness, was also important. This includes not only physical attractiveness but also an agreeable and warm personality. Collette (1969) found that when he asked dentists about their ideal patients, they replied that they should be well educated, at the upper end of the socioeconomic scale and between 25 and 55 years of age—just the kind of patients who could be expected to be manageable, treatable and attractive.

It is interesting to speculate on the relationship between attendance, socioeconomic status and the interpersonal aspects of care. There is a well established association between socioeconomic status and attendance patterns, but this does not seem to be due to economic factors alone (see Chapter 1). Since dentists are of a high socioeconomic level, they would be expected to relate well with high-status patients. This could account for why, for these patients, the technical competence of the dentist is paramount—they relate well to most dentists with few difficulties. On the other hand, patients of lower socioeconomic status will have more difficulties with their dentists, perhaps explaining why they put priority on reassurance and friendliness. This kind of reasoning has led some researchers to argue that the low utilization rates of some patients is due to their dissatisfaction with the interpersonal aspects of dental care.

Negative stereotypes

This argument is supported by the finding that some dentists have negative stereotypes of patients from low educational and economic backgrounds. Frazier et al. (1977) developed a short description of a patient, called 'Mrs D', who was said to have had only a few years of formal education, who was divorced with five children and who was dependent on government agencies for her income. The dentists were then asked about their expectations of Mrs D. In one question, they were asked to rank in order which goods and services she would be most likely to want. The alternatives were 'a good car', 'education', 'nice clothes', 'dental care' and a 'colour TV or stereo'. The dentists believed that she would order her priorities in the following order: nice clothes, colour TV, good car, dental care and education. Then Frazier et al. interviewed a group of mothers who were in many ways similar to Mrs D, asking them to rank their actual priorities. Very different results were found. For them, their priorities were education first, then dental care, nice clothes, a good car and finally the colour TV.

Just what effects such stereotypes have on patient care is not known, but they may affect care in two ways. First, there may be some under-utilization of services by people who feel that their problems and values are not recognized by dentists. As indicated earlier, most irregular attenders place most emphasis on reassurance and friendliness, while it seems likely that most dentists would emphasize technical skill. A second—more controversial—possibility is that they might be given poorer technical care. This latter possibility has been given some limited support by Weinstein et al. (1979) who found that patients who were well motivated and co-operative—qualities which are valued by most dentists—received somewhat better care, as measured by the quality of restorations. There is more support for this notion in other areas of patient care, where several studies have shown that health care professionals prefer, spend more time with and have more success with patients who are similar to themselves and share their values (Berkanovic and Reeder, 1974; Wills, 1978).

Communication

These studies illustrate the point that dental care is two-way, in that both dentist and patient contribute to outcome. Szasz and Hollender (1956) have described three types of relationship which can occur between professional care-givers and patients. One is termed *activity–passivity*, where the professional is in complete active control and the patient is a passive recipient of treatment. In dentistry, this type of relationship could occur when the patient is under a general anaesthetic. A second type of relationship is *guidance–co-operation*, when the professional guides (like a teacher) while the patient co-operates (like a student). This seems to describe the situation where the dentist is treating a conscious patient—typically, the dentist will indicate the work which needs to be done and the patient will agree. The third type is termed *mutual participation*. It is most clearly shown in preventive care, where the dentist and patient share responsibility for the maintenance of oral health (Ayer, 1982).

Involving the patient in treatment decisions

There is no one kind of relationship which is appropriate for all situations. On some occasions one will be appropriate while on other occasions another will be required. It seems likely that problems will arise if there is a mismatch between the expectations of the dentist and those of the patient, where one individual is working under one approach while the other believes a different kind of relationship is called for. To take the fitting of dentures as an example, Lefer et al. (1962) note that one view in dentistry is that patients should be persuaded to choose appliances which complement their personality and appearance, and any resistance shown by the patient should be overcome. According to this view, the dentist is in the best position to make this aesthetic decision and any resistance to the dentist's choice should be overcome for the patient's own good. Lefer et al. argue that this approach is seriously misplaced since it relies on the professional's view of what is right for the patient, a view which might not be shared by the patient him- or herself.

Lefer et al. performed a simple experiment to test the hypothesis that patients would be more satisfied with their dentures if they were involved in the choice. One group of dentists were asked to treat their patients in the normal fashion, which was usually deciding themselves on the dentures' appearance. The other dentists were instructed to involve the patients in the choice: the patients were asked to select the size, colour and set-up of the appliance from 12 possibilities. The dentists told the patients to 'Take your time until you come to your own decision' and 'Your opinion is more important than mine'. It soon became clear that the dentists' choices did not correspond particularly well with the patients'. For example, over 50% of the patients given a choice preferred a 'textbook' set-up, but this was given by the dentists in the no-choice group to only 15% of the patients. By contrast, the type of denture given by the dentists 50% of the time was chosen by only 30% of the patients. On average, those given a choice required only half as many adjustments (mean = 1.5) than those given no choice (mean = 2.9). They were less likely to complain or reject the appliance and made fewer visits for corrections.

In general, patients seemed to prefer set-ups which were similar to their natural teeth. Patients who had the decision made for them made comments like 'I wish they were a little darker and longer—the way my own teeth used to look', while patients who were given the right to choose expressed their satisfaction (e.g. 'That's how I wanted to look and I've been happy with the results').

The dentist's personality

This study indicated that involving the patient in the choice of dentures resulted in fewer complaints. However, involvement itself may not be adequate since the personality of the dentist can also affect satisfaction. In another study (Hirsch et al., 1973) dental students were given a personality questionnaire designed to measure authoritarianism, which is a personality trait referring to the extent to which a person is power-oriented in relationships. Someone who scores high on authoritarianism tends to be obedient to those considered superior, but dominant over those seen as inferior. The students were then asked to construct an appliance which their patients had previously been involved in selecting. At the end of the treatment a faculty member examined the dentures to be sure that they were clinically satisfactory and that the patients' wishes had been followed. The interest was in the relationship between the students' scores on the authoritarianism questionnaire and patient ratings of the dentures.

As shown in Fig. 7.1, the patients were asked to give a rating of their choice both before and after it was constructed: before treatment the patients gave ratings between 'good' and 'very good', but after treatment

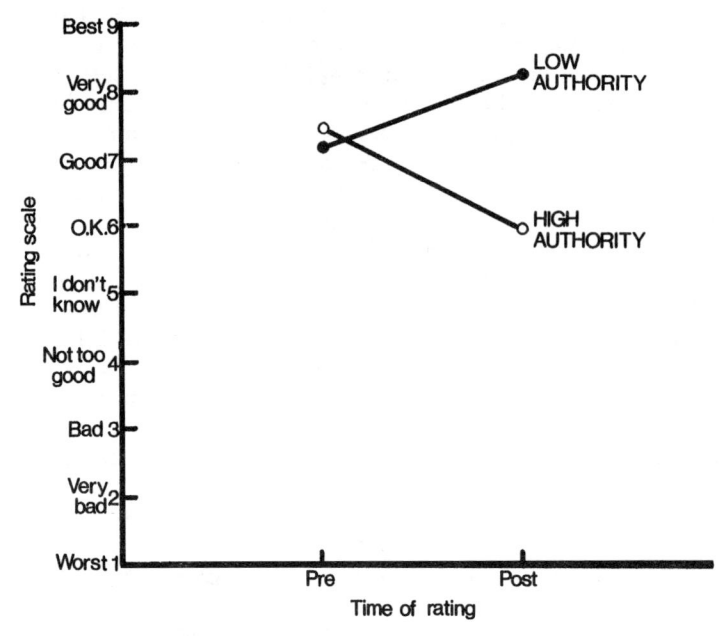

Figure 7.1 Patients' ratings of denture set-ups before and after they were constructed by high- and low-authoritarian students. From Hirsch et al. (1973), with permission.

there was a significant difference between those assigned to high- and low-authoritarian students. The patients in the former group now reported less satisfaction than those in the latter group. This was not due to the high-authoritarian students being less capable clinically since the dentures were all passed as satisfactory by the staff. It seemed that the students' personalities affected satisfaction in some way.

Patients' complaints
Unfortunately, there was no follow-up of these patients, so it is not possible to gauge the long-term consequences of authoritarianism. It would also have been useful to have made a recording of the consultations between students and patients so that the different ways the high- and low-authoritarian students related to their patients could have been specified. However, an analysis of letters of complaint sent to a dental society supports the idea that the willingness of a dentist to listen, negotiate and share responsibility with a patient is important. For example:

> The reason I went to . . . is because I thought I would get my teeth done the way I wanted them done. He had long white teeth in the impression set so I told him I'd like smaller teeth and my face filled out a bit more. He became angry and said it would be better to have the pink part thin, and he didn't want to use small teeth and said they wouldn't be right for my age. I said I'd still prefer to have smaller teeth and my face filled out more, but he became annoyed and walked out of the room. The nurse came in and dismissed me.

and:

The reason I asked ... to replace the cap on my front tooth was to improve my appearance, and I made that quite clear from the start. I told him I wanted the tooth a certain shape. Also, I wanted the tooth smooth, the same shade all over, as the old cap had a yellow splotch. When he first put in the new cap, I told him it was too narrow at the neck and not straight as it slanted towards the centre. He replied that it was natural to slant that way and his did. Then I showed him that the bottom half of the cap was blue. He said this was done because it looked more natural this way. He knew I wasn't happy about the cap but how can I get anywhere with him as he is always right and I am always wrong? (Hirsch et al., 1973, pp. 747–748).

In order to provide guidelines for the practitioner, a detailed examination of communication patterns between dentist and patient could be very useful. Once some general patterns have been established these could be elaborated and refined by the practitioner for use with individual patients.

Verbal communication

One of the more important studies in this area was conducted by Wurster et al. (1979). They examined the communication patterns between senior dental students and their child patients. The appointments were recorded on videotape and the students' and patients' behaviour later noted: every 6 seconds a judge rated the kind of behaviour being shown at that moment. For the children, behaviour was rated as being co-operative (responding in a relaxed and non-fearful manner), resistant (when the child seemed to be experiencing some distress but this was not interfering with treatment) or unco-operative (resistance to the point of interfering with treatment). The students' behaviour was categorized as being directive and guiding (e.g. providing a straightforward statement of instruction while encouraging the patient), permissive (allowing any disruptive behaviour to continue unabated) or coercive (attempting to overcome disruption by threatening, ridiculing or using physical restraint). Then, Wurster et al. examined the tapes to see how the children reacted (co-operative, resistant or unco-operative) to each of the different actions (guidance, permissiveness or coercion) shown by the students. Results indicated a 0.85 probability that direction and guidance would be followed by co-operation, a 0.67 probability that permissiveness would be followed by non-co-operation and a 0.97 probability that coerciveness would be followed by non-co-operation or resistance.

It is not, however, possible to say from this study that direction and guidance lead to or cause co-operation because the child may have been co-operating to begin with and the students were responding to this. In other words, the students may have been reacting to the children, rather than vice versa. This interpretation is supported by the results of a further analysis of the tapes where the communication patterns were examined from the other direction, looking to see what the students did after co-operation, resistance or non-co-operation. When the children were co-operative, the students almost always responded by directive guidance (probability = 0.93), but when the child behaved in an unco-operative manner the students usually responded by permissive or coercive behaviour (probability = 0.73).

In order to say that certain behaviour on the part of the dentist leads to certain behaviour on the part of the child patient it would be necessary to examine those instances when a child is being disruptive, look at how the dentist reacts, and then relate this to the child's subsequent behaviour. Do different kinds of reactions result in different kinds of behaviour? Weinstein et al. (1982) used this method in their study of dentists and their child patients. All the children were 3–5 years of age, having appointments for routine treatment. At each point in time their behaviour was categorized as being either fearful (as shown by, for example, crying, movement or protest) or non-fearful. When they were showing fearful behaviour the dentists' responses were noted and the probability that these would be followed by continuing fear was computed. At such times, the probability that continued fearful behaviour would continue was 0.82 when the dentist was coercive, 0.55 when the dentist was coaxing and 0.48 when the dentist set specific rules for behaviour. When the dentist belittled or ignored the child the probabilities of fearful behaviour continuing were also high. By contrast, when the dentist questioned the children about their feelings, or asked rhetorical questions, fearful behaviour decreased (probabilities of 0.37 and 0.26). Explanation and direction (0.30 and 0.20 respectively) were useful responses. When the dentist gave praise, specific comments like 'I like the way you keep your mouth open' were more effective than general ones, like 'Good boy' (Weinstein and Nathan, 1988). The dentist's non-verbal behaviour was also important, as discussed below.

Experimental methods can be used to examine the effects of dentists' behaviour on their patients, by asking dentists to react in certain ways to disruptive or unco-operative behaviour. There is some preliminary work using this approach, where it was found that those children who were reprimanded for inappropriate or disruptive behaviour showed the most anxiety but when the dentist was more neutral and unevaluative the greatest degree of compliant behaviour was shown (Melamed et al., 1983).

Non-verbal communication

These studies indicate that some kinds of response to disruptive behaviour are more effective than others. However, everything a dentist says is embedded within a frame of non-verbal behaviour which serves to elaborate and modify the meaning of a statement. Generally speaking, the non-verbal aspects of conversation have a greater impact on the emotional quality of relationships, whereas verbal communication is more relevant to shared cognitive tasks and problems. Indications of friendship, assertiveness and dominance, for example, seem to depend more on non-verbal than verbal behaviour (Argyle, 1969; Argyle et al., 1972).

There are a great many non-verbal signals which influence our interactions with other people. Even the architectural features of the dentist's office can convey many messages. Besides the general décor of an office, there may be architectural barriers which prevent some patients from receiving the services they need. A narrow door, a surgery which is not large enough to accommodate a wheelchair or a great many steps are non-verbal indications that physically handicapped people have not been considered. During conversation, the way we sit, move and look are some important influences, as are the context of the encounter and the nature of past interactions. For example, eye gaze can have two distinct and almost incompatible meanings, depending on the circumstances. When two people know each other well and the circumstances are friendly, long periods of looking at each other suggest intimacy, but when issues of status are at hand, eye gaze may indicate aggression. Similarly, touching may indicate caring or dominance.

Furthermore, many non-verbal signals interact with each other. Argyle and Ingram (1972) reported that people look at each other more frequently when they are separated by a large distance than when they are close together. They suggest that eye gaze and distance can substitute for each other as signs of intimacy, so that in order to keep a constant level of intimacy people will look at each other less often and for shorter periods of time when they are close together. An everyday example of this can be found in crowded buses—everyone is standing close together and studiously looking out of the window or at the advertisements.

Vision
Being able to see a conversational partner is not necessary for interaction (it is possible, for instance, to talk over the telephone) but it does play an important role in most conversations. When a person is speaking, he or she will tend to look at the partner infrequently and for short periods of time, presumably because of a concern with formulating what to say. Attention is mainly focused on thinking. However, speakers do look at their partners occasionally, apparently to gain information as to whether they are being understood. It is during these times that listeners provide feedback, nodding their heads and murmuring agreement. When a person is listening, he or she will spend most of the time looking at the speaker, showing attention to what is being said. Listeners who do not look and who do not nod their heads are often judged to be unfriendly and uninterested in the speaker. Whether speaking or listening, the amount of gaze a person gives appears to affect others' perceptions of friendliness and warmth. Thus, a patient who is visually ignored by the dentist may well feel that the dentist is not especially warm or caring.

While there appear to be no studies in the dental literature relating eye gaze to patients' behaviour or satisfaction with their care, there are several studies concerned with its role in doctor–patient consultations. For example, Byrne and Heath (1980) videotaped several interviews, looking especially at the relationship between doctors' behaviour and the speaking patterns of the patients. Clearly, the patients would stop speaking—sometimes in mid-sentence—whenever the doctor looked down and began writing. Only when the doctor looked up again did the patients resume. Apparently, the patients assumed that the doctors were attending to their writing and would not be listening to what they said.

The reader may be interested in testing these ideas with his or her own patients. It could be useful to note if they stop describing their symptoms or difficulties when you appear to be busy with some other task.

Posture and gestures
The posture assumed by conversationalists is very important. A slight forward lean has been shown to be associated with perceptions of warmth. Closed-arm positions appear to indicate coldness or rejection while moderately open arm positions convey warmth and acceptance. Changes in posture can convey a wealth of information. They often accompany a change in topic and can be used to signal the end of a conversation. If people are seated while talking, for instance, when one participant stands up the aim is often to finish the conversation. Movement is also used to emphasize a point or to demonstrate an idea. The representation of size with the hands commonly occurs: people often hold them far apart when describing a large object, close together when describing something small. Facial movements comprise perhaps the most expressive non-verbal signals. Many are common to all cultures, since people of very different upbringings smile, laugh and cry in similar ways.

Posture, gestures and facial movements are some non-verbal signals which are commonly used to infer patients' anxiety or pain, but as discussed in earlier chapters the correlations between dentists' ratings of overt behaviour and patients' self-reports of anxiety and pain are by no means perfect, and often quite low. This may be because there is, in fact, little relationship between the two or, alternatively, that not all dentists are particularly skilled at discerning inner feelings from overt behaviour. There is evidence from the medical literature that some doctors are much more adept than others in their ability to appreciate the emotions of patients, a point taken up later in the chapter.

Proximity
One way of understanding the distance that people keep between each other is in terms of 'personal space'—a kind of bubble of portable territory. A method of discovering the size of this space is simply to observe conversationalists and then measure the distance between them. When standing or talking casually, people in our culture usually keep about 2–2½ ft between them. In other cultures the distance is smaller. A way of testing the validity of this observation is simply to walk closer to someone and measure the distance at which he or she begins to move backwards. The point at which this occurs is the edge of the bubble. It seems from experiments of this type that the bubble is not round: people will tolerate more proximity at their sides than at the front or back.

The boundaries of personal space vary according to several situational factors. Intimacy of topic is one variable, as is the relationship between the participants (e.g. friends or strangers). Hall (1967) categorized proximity into four zones: intimate (0–18 in), personal (18 in to 4 ft), social (4–12 ft) and public (more than 12 ft). The topic of conversation and the relationship between the participants using these different zones vary. For instance, two people standing or sitting between 4 and 12 ft apart are more likely to be speaking socially than personally or intimately.

Much dental care involves the intimate zone, particularly physical contact. Weinstein et al. (1982), in their study of the effects of dentists' behaviour on the fear of their child patients discussed earlier, assessed the probabilities of continuing fear following various forms of touching. Holding and restraining increased the likelihood of fearful responses (probability 0.62 and 0.85 respectively), while patting seemed to reduce it (probability = 0.30).

It is also interesting to speculate on the meaning of an oral examination and treatment for patients in this regard. Like doctors and nurses, dentists seem to have a kind of special licence to enter personal space and touch patients, but there is little evidence to indicate whether this results in uncomfortable feelings or whether patients feel completely neutral about it. Simply because it is culturally acceptable for dentists to touch their patients cannot be taken as an indication that there are no significant meanings attached. Nurses also have the right to touch their patients but they often find them disclosing very personal information during intimate forms of touching. Medical patients sometimes complain that they feel violated in some way when doctors physically examine them without any prior attempt to establish some rapport. Because of the link between touch and intimacy, it may be important that dentists, too, spend some time with a new patient before attempting examination in order to develop an appropriate relationship.

Teaching communication skills

Perhaps the most frequent question asked about the training of communication skills is: Why are they needed? Every dentist is, after all, a highly skilled psychologist in many ways, having had much experience with many people. Many of the abilities needed should be 'picked up' during the dental course by watching how members of staff relate to their patients and later by noting how patients react to comments and advice. While there is some validity in these arguments, there are also indications that this kind of informal training is not always adequate. In the training of medical students there is an awareness that the emphasis placed on technical skills has left an important gap in their education. For example, Helfer (1970) compared the interviewing skills of senior medical students with those of students just entering the medical course. He found that the senior students fared worse at eliciting important problems besides those presented directly by the patients themselves. While the senior students were more adept at assessing the patients' medical condition, they obtained less information about relevant personal difficulties than did the new students, suggesting that medical training restricted the students' outlook and actually had a detrimental effect on some interviewing skills. In another study (Maguire and Rutter, 1976), one-third of the senior students failed to elicit the patient's main illness or problem and psychological and social aspects of the illness were commonly neglected. On average, they obtained only one-quarter of the information an independent judge considered relevant and easily obtainable.

In response to such findings, most medical schools now include some communication skills training in their curricula. There are indications that similar programmes would also be useful for dental students. In their study of students and child patients outlined earlier, Wurster et al. (1979) asked the students to rate their confidence in their ability to cope with difficult patients. The students were given a series of hypothetical situations, such as: 'Four-year-old Donna attempts to leave the chair during placement of a rubber dam'. They were asked to indicate their ability to cope with such situations on a 10-point scale ranging between 'I feel my skills are disturbingly inadequate. I do not think I am able to control this behaviour more than one time out of 10' and 'I feel my skills are completely adequate. I am able to control this behaviour whenever it occurs'. The students were then divided into high- and low-confidence groups and their behaviour with the patients noted. The less confident students accounted for 86% of the permissive behaviours and 95% of the coercive ones. As discussed earlier, these were the kinds of reactions associated with unco-operative behaviour on the part of the children and, indeed, the patients of the less confident students accounted for 87% of the unco-operative behaviour shown by all the children in the study. Since the children were assigned to students without knowledge of their confidence level, it seems unlikely that this difference was due to the children's personalities.

It is useful to consider interpersonal abilities as particular kinds of skills, much like riding a bicycle, driving a car or drilling a cavity. When first learning to drive, a person may feel awkward and unsure, but soon becomes more comfortable as the skills become automatic. A student who is about to drill his or her first cavity on a patient is likely to be anxious and unsteady, but with practice the action becomes more assured and smooth. Just as these physical skills can be taught and developed, so too can social skills. Many programmes have been developed coming under the rubric of 'social skills training' (SST; Furnham, 1983). This approach has been used in a variety of situations from helping managers to communicate with their employees to helping doctors in their consultations with patients. Some dental schools include social skills training in their curricula, and examples of these programmes are discussed next.

Training programmes

One of the most important concepts in patient care of almost any type is called 'accurate empathy'. This refers to two complementary abilities. The first involves the ability to discern the meaning of patients' verbal and non-verbal behaviour. The second component is the ability to express the understanding gained through this sensitivity. That is, it is not only important to be able to gauge emotions but also to indicate this to the patient. Research in medical care has indicated that doctors possess these abilities to different degrees and that they are related to patients' feelings of being listened to and understood and their wish to see the same doctor again (DiMatteo et al., 1979, 1980).

Such results could be expected to apply to dentist–patient relationships as well and there are several programmes which attempt to increase dentists' accurate empathy. Jackson (1975, 1978b) describes his approach in some detail. He argues that many of the comments made by dental patients have both a surface and a deeper, more subtle meaning. For example, a patient could say to a dentist who is new to a practice: 'I liked . . . I went to him for 30 years, you know', or a parent could say: 'Can I come into the surgery with my son?'. In his training programme he encourages students to *translate* such comments, looking for alternative meanings. So in the first example the possibility that the patient is saying 'I'm not sure that I trust you' might be considered, or in the second example perhaps the parent is saying 'I am worried about my son's dental care and whether you will treat him properly'. Jackson suggests that statements referring to the amount of work required, length of treatment, size of cavity and necessity for a local anaesthetic probably reflect fears of discomfort, while comments about the equipment, age of the dentist and difficulty of the procedures frequently represent patients' concerns with technical competence.

Types of response

The next step involves a consideration of how the students might respond to such comments. First, a distinction is made between relevant and irrelevant responses, so that

Patient: I see you have a new drill.
Dentist: Yes, a Siemens 242 x 43, a real beauty.

would be considered an irrelevant response, since it is unlikely that the patient was concerned about the name of the equipment, more likely that he was expressing some degree of anxiety about it.

Relevant responses fall into four categories:

1 *Evaluative responses,* which tend to make patients feel that they are being evaluated negatively or told that they should not feel the way they do, e.g.:

Patient: I brush my teeth and floss at least once a day and I think it is ridiculous that I have two cavities this check-up.
Dentist: Now, I never gave you any assurances that you wouldn't still have some cavities; anyway, two small cavities is a pretty good check-up. You should be very satisfied.

When this exchange is translated, it might read:

Patient: I am disappointed and frustrated.
Dentist: I do not approve of you being disappointed and frustrated. You should be very satisfied.

Another example:

Patient (a child): I hate dentists. I don't want to be here. I want to go home.

Dentist: Come now. Even your little brother didn't mind his check-up. Be a good boy and open your mouth.

This could be translated as

Patient: I am afraid.
Dentist: Because you are afraid I think you are both childish and bad.

2 *Supportive responses,* which imply that it is unnecessary for the patient to feel as he does, e.g.:

Patient: I am really concerned about this extraction.
Dentist: No need to be, it does not seem to be a very difficult one. It should not take more than 10 minutes.

3 *Probing responses* ask for more information or explanation. It is useful to use the patient's own words if possible, e.g.:

Patient: I hate going to the dentist.
Dentist: What do you hate about it?

4 *Understanding responses,* which indicate that the dentist realizes and accepts the patient's concern, e.g.:

Patient: Can I come into the surgery with my son?
Dentist: You're wondering how he will react.

Such training programmes make the assumption that it is in some way better for a dentist to act in an understanding or supportive way than to be evaluative or irrelevant. In order to test this asumption, Jackson gave examples of written conversations between dentists and patients to (non-dental) students, so that, for example, all the students saw the patient's comment:

> The only reason I'm here is because this tooth is killing me, otherwise you'd never find me in a dentist's chair.

but one-third saw the evaluative response:

> If you would have come in for regular check-ups, you probably would not be having so much pain.

another third saw the supportive response:

> Don't worry, we'll look after you.

and the rest the understanding one:

> It really bothers you to see the dentist.

The students were shown several such conversations and asked to make judgements about the kinds of dentists who would make such responses. The understanding and supportive dentists were said to be significantly more sensitive, altruistic and warm than the evaluative ones.

Programme evaluation

It is important to evaluate training programmes in order to measure their effectiveness. Such evaluation could be conducted by comparing students' behaviour before and after a training course or by giving the course to one group of students while another group, not given the training, serves as a comparison. Jackson used the latter approach. Half the students were given a course of three 2-h sessions describing the ideas of attending and responding, as described above. Students in the control group received no training in these ideas. Then, all were asked to role-play a dentist who was to explain the reasons for an extraction to someone who was playing the role of a patient. This patient did not want the treatment. Their consultation was videotaped and later shown to two judges who rated the students' behaviour on a number of dimensions, including empathy, respect and genuineness. These were not the specific skills taught but, rather, more global assessments of interpersonal ability and warmth. When the ratings of the two groups of students were compared, those given the training programme were seen to be significantly more able, particularly on the scales of empathy and respect.

Another kind of training programme is described by Levy et al. (1980). The students were first given a 1-h overview of the content of the course. A brief description of 12 patient management skills was provided. These included many of the ideas discussed in earlier chapters, such as giving positive reinforcement for co-operative behaviour, the importance of providing truthful and accurate information and informing patients that they could raise their arms whenever they wished to say something or to indicate discomfort. Then, each student was observed during an appointment with a patient. The observer noted two kinds of behaviour (e.g. information giving and positive reinforcement) which seemed lacking for each student. These deficits were then discussed and the students were to try to improve them during subsequent appointments. When the students' behaviour in one of these subsequent appointments was monitored, there was a significant improvement in the behaviour previously discussed.

Gaining feedback
One problem that dentists face is in knowing if a consultation has succeeded or not from the patient's point of view. Few patients express dissatisfaction to their dentists directly. It is more probable that they will simply go elsewhere for their next appointment. This leaves the dentist not knowing if the patient has moved away, is content but has not attended for a long time, or has found another dentist. Some methods for increasing feedback have already been mentioned, such as asking

probing questions and using non-verbal signs of interest. Some training programmes have included a formal feedback process. During training, a student might be asked to videotape a consultation with a patient and then to play the tape back in the presence of peers or staff. In some programmes, the patients themselves are also present at the play-back, so that they can contribute their viewpoint. By asking both patients and students to discuss the thoughts they had during the interview a more complete understanding of the consultation can be achieved (Kent et al., 1981).

This can, however, be expensive in time and Gershen et al. (1980) have developed an interesting alternative. They first videotaped some appointments between dentists and their patients. Then, each dentist and patient and a member of the dental school teaching staff discussed the tape in depth. This conversation was in turn audiotaped and the participants' comments edited on to the original videotape. This meant that the appointments could be shown to dental students with both the dentist's and patient's comments being included in the background. While this method has the disadvantage of not being tailored to each student's requirements, it is a readily available teaching aid for calling attention to the patient's feelings and concerns during treatment.

Stress in dentistry

Dentistry has something of a reputation for being a particularly stressful occupation. However comparisons between dentists and other health professionals indicate that they do not have an appreciably higher prevalence of morbidity; other people have physical and psychological problems too. A high rate of suicide is a widely quoted statistic, but in fact the research on this is based on extremely small numbers and cannot be considered reliable (Kent, 1987). Some studies have shown a lower rate than expected for age and race (Dean, 1969; Hill and Harvey, 1972).

Sources of stress

This is not to say that dentistry is stress-free. When Godwin et al. (1981) asked recent graduates to describe 'the sources of greatest stress', 73% mentioned patient management (which included some reference to patient fear and anxiety, late or missed appointments and patient dissatisfaction with their services), 50% mentioned business management problems (such as collection of fees, cash-flow problems, overheads and insurance), and 38% indicated that their own perfectionism led to frustration due to the discrepancy between their high ideals for care and the realities of day-to-day dentistry. Problems with staff management were cited by 33%, and 26% indicated that time pressures, particularly when they fell behind schedule, were a source of stress.

Clearly it is not easy being a private dental practitioner. There is also some work on the incidence of major problems, such as the death of a patient under general anaesthetic or other serious reactions to drugs. In Young's (1975) survey, 43% of the dentists had experienced at least one occasion within the previous 5 years when resuscitation was necessary. While the incidence for specific problems was low (e.g. for respiratory arrest it was 0.02 cases per dentist per year), the average practitioner may worry about his or her ability to respond appropriately should an emergency occur. Such a concern was illustrated by one dentist who claimed that he had given a large number of general anaesthetics over the past 10 years without trouble, but added the rider 'so something has to happen soon'.

Stress in specialties
Despite the general finding that dentistry does not lead to greater morbidity than other health professions, dentists in some specialties appear to be more at risk than others. Coronary heart disease is one problem commonly associated with stress. Russek (1962) posted questionnaires to dentists in four specialties which were considered to involve varying levels of stressfulness—general practice (most), oral surgery, orthodontics and periodontology (least). After the results were adjusted for age, there was a gradation in the number of heart complaints reported by the dentists, with those in general practice reporting almost three times the incidence of coronary heart disease than those in periodontology. Whether these differences were due solely to the relative stressfulness of the specialties or partly influenced by self-selection into the specialties cannot be ascertained from this study. It may be that the kinds of dentists who choose general practice or oral surgery are more prone to heart disease than those who choose orthodontics or periodontology. This is an important possibility to consider because there are indications that some doctors who select general medical practice (a specialty in medicine which is associated with a high risk for coronaries) are more vulnerable to stress-related illnesses (Vaillant et al., 1972).

Stress in dental school
The stresses reported by students depend to some extent on their year of the course, but academic concerns relating to the volume of material (rather than with conceptual difficulty) are generally rated highly. Inconsistent feedback from staff is often a problem (Goldstein, 1979). Sachs et al. (1981) identified several concerns. These included relationships with teachers (e.g. 'being treated as though you were immature and irresponsible' and 'dealing with authoritarian, unsympathetic instructors'), academic worries (e.g. 'being unable to learn everything' and 'fear of making a mistake'), feeling lonely, and financial troubles.

Recognition that such problems are widespead amongst dentists and dental students can itself be reassuring. It is 'normal' for students to be anxious when treating patients, or for experienced dentists to be concerned about the possibility of a medical emergency (Cooper et al., 1987). It is common for health professionals to believe that they *should* be able to cope with their professional lives with little difficulty and may feel ashamed if they cannot. This belief often inhibits individuals from discussing their problems with others. The relief experienced when someone discovers that their difficulties are being experienced by colleagues can be profound.

Stress management

The training in communication skills mentioned earlier in the chapter can help to reduce stress. Not only does training benefit the dentist–patient relationship, it also increases confidence and ability to handle difficult situations. The same principles apply to relationships with staff as well. However there are several other more direct ways to reduce stress. O'Shea et al. (1984) found that practising dentists used a variey of strategies, including exercise, taking time off work, and hobbies. Although such methods are effective in the short run, they involve avoiding, rather than attempting to change, the situation. The programme advocated by Bosmajian and Bosmajian (1983) provides a structured approach to change. They argue that stress can only be reduced if an individual is first aware of those situations which cause stress. To this end, they provide a 'stresslog'. The dentist is encouraged to note the situations where stress occurs, what the events imply, and what responses were made. The completion of such a diary allows the dentist to see repeating patterns in both events and responses.

Once a detailed record is made over several weeks a pattern may emerge. The stresslog may indicate that you are frequently frustrated by the quality of your work due to time pressures. This could be related to some of the erroneous assumptions which dentists often make about their practice, such as those suggested by Ireland (1983):

1 I should be appreciated by every patient.
2 To be worthwhile, I must be thoroughly competent and successful in my field.
3 I should be emotionally concerned for every patient.
4 There is always a right, precise and perfect solution to a patient's problems, and this solution must always be found.

Having such high and unrealistic expectations about one's own performance will almost certainly result in stress when these standards cannot be met.

Alternatively, a dentist may find that the stressful situations often involve relationships with other members of the dental team. The acquisition of effective management skills (Emling, 1980) is important here, especially since Locker et al. (1989) found that one of the main sources of dental assistants' stress was feeling undervalued by the dentist. Students may identify a completely different set of stressors. For some it could be a lack of confidence in dealing with patients while for others it could be anxiety about the workload. Some dental schools provide workshops in study skills and encourage small group discussions where problems can be aired, strategies for studying shared and emotional support given (Schwartz et al., 1984). (Appendix 1 provides some tips on studying.) Stress management programmes have been evaluated and shown to be effective (Tisdelle et al., 1984).

Summary

While most research relating psychology to dentistry has concerned patients, the personal qualities and behaviour of the dentist are also significant. The strength of the placebo effect in reducing pain, for instance, is related to the warmth and enthusiasm of the dentist. When patients are asked which characteristics are most important in a dentist, technical competence is given first priority followed by such personality characteristics as warmth, being reassuring and 'putting you at your ease'. Patients of high socioeconomic status and regular attenders often place technical skill first, but those of low socioeconomic status and irregular attenders give most emphasis to the interpersonal aspects of care.

Communication involves both verbal and non-verbal behaviour. While coercion, coaxing and belittling patients increases disruption, explanation and direction serve to increase co-operation. The words spoken by a dentist are embedded within a large number of non-verbal signals, such as eye gaze, proximity and gestures. These non-verbal signs have a strong influence on the meaning of verbal messages. They, too, can affect co-operation: for example, gently patting a patient can reduce fearful behaviour while restraint seems to increase it.

One of the more important personal qualities needed by health care professionals is called 'accurate empathy', which involves both the ability to understand what patients mean by their verbal and non-verbal communication and the ability to express this understanding to them. Some dental schools include training programmes in their curricula which are designed to improve these abilities, sometimes through direct instruction and sometimes by observation of students' behaviour with patients.

Practice implications

1 Patients extrapolate from their personal experiences with a dentist to beliefs about technical competence. When building and maintaining a practice, special care needs to be given to developing relationships with patients.
2 Since satisfaction is a result of both emotional (trust) and cognitive (understanding) factors, it is important that patients are given time to express their concerns and to ask questions.
3 Making tape recordings of consultations (with the consent of patients and other staff) and reviewing these with colleagues is a powerful way of increasing social skills.
4 General practice is a stressful way of making a living for many dentists. Keeping a 'stress' diary may allow you to pinpoint difficult situations and provide clues as to how to change them.

Suggested reading

DiMatteo M.R. and DiNicola D.A. *Achieving Patient Compliance* (Oxford, Pergamon, 1982) provides a comprehensive review of the literature concerning doctor–patient communication. A useful overview of stress management for dentists is Christen A.G., McDonald J. (eds) *Management of Stress in the Dental Practitioner. The Dental Clinics of North America (suppl.).* (London, Saunders, 1986).

References

Abrams R.A., Ayers C., Petterson M. (1986) Quality assessment of dental restorations: a comparison by dentists and patients. *Community Dent. Oral. Epidemiol.* **14**, 317-19.
Argyle M. (1969) *Social Interaction*. London: Methuen.
Argyle M., Ingram R. (1972) Gaze, mutual gaze and proximity. *Semiotica* **6**, 32-44.
Argyle M., Alkema F., Gilmour R. (1972) The communication of friendly and hostile attitudes by verbal and non-verbal signals. *Eur. J. Soc. Psychol.* **1**, 385-402.
Ayer W. A. (1982) The dentist-patient relationship. *Int. Dent. J.* **32**, 56-64.
Ben-Sira Z. (1982) Lay evaluation of medical treatment and competence: development of a model of the function of the physician's affective behaviour. *Soc. Sci. Med.* **16**, 1013-19.
Berkanovic E., Reeder L. G. (1974) Can money buy the appropriate use of services? Some notes on the meaning of utilisation data. *J. Health Soc. Behav.* **15**, 93-9.
Bosmajian C.P., Bosmajian L. (1983) *Personalised Guide to Stress Evaluation*. London: Mosby.
Bulman J. S., Richard N. D., Slack G. C. et al. (1968) *Demand and Need for Dental Care*. London: Oxford University Press.
Byrne P. S., Heath C. C. (1980) Practitioner's use of non-verbal behaviour in real consultations. *J. R. Coll. Gen. Pract.* **30**, 327-31.
Collette H. A. (1969) Influence of dentist-patient relationships on attitudes and adjustments to dental treatment. *J. Am. Dent. Assoc.* **79**, 879-84.
Cooper C.L., Watts J., Kelly M. (1987) Job satisfaction, mental health and job stressors among general dental practitioners in the UK. *Br. Dent. J.* **162**, 77-81.
Dean G. (1969) The causes of death of South African doctors and dentists. *South Afr. Med. J.* **43**, 495-500.
DiMatteo M. R., Friedman H. S., Taranta A. (1979) Sensitivity to bodily non-verbal communication as a factor in practitioner-patient rapport. *J. Nonverb. Behav.* **4**, 18-26.
DiMatteo M. R., Taranta A., Friedman H. S. et al. (1980) Predicting patient satisfaction from physicians' non-verbal communication skills. *Med. Care* **18**, 376-87.
Emling R.C. (1980) Employee and patient management in times of stress. *Compend. Cont. Educ. Dent.* **1**, 351-5.
Frazier P. J., Jenny J., Bagramian R. A. et al. (1977) Provider expectations and consumer perceptions of the importance and value of dental care. *Am J. Public Health* **67**, 37-43.
Furnham A. (1983) Social skills and dentistry. *Br. Dent. J.* **154**, 404-8.
Garfunkel E. (1980) The consumer speaks: how patients select and how much they know about dental health care personnel. *J. Prosthet. Dent.* **43**, 380-4.
Gershen J. A., Marcus M., Strohlein A. et al. (1980) An application of interpersonal process recall for teaching behavioural science in dentistry. *J. Dent. Educ.* **44**, 268-9.
Godwin W.C., Starks D., Green T., Koran A. (1981) Identification of sources of stress in practice by recent dental graduates. *J. Dent. Educ.* **45**, 220-1.
Goldstein M.B. (1979) Sources of stress and interpersonal support among first year dental students. *J. Dent. Educ.* **43**, 625-9.
Gryll S. L., Katahn H. (1978) Situational factors contributing to the placebo effect. *Psychopharmacol.* **57**, 253-61.
Hall E. T. (1967) *The Hidden Dimension*. London: Bodley Head.
Helfer R. C. (1970) An objective comparison of the paediatric interviewing skills of freshmen and senior medical students. *Paediatrics* **45**, 623-7.
Hengst A., Roghmann K. (1978) The two dimensions in satisfaction with dental care. *Medical Care,* **16**, 202-10.
Hill G.B., Harvey W. (1972) Mortality of dentists. *Br. Dent. J.* **132**, 179-82.
Hirsch B., Levine B., Tiber N. (1973) Effects of dentist authoritarianism on patient evaluation of dentures. *J. Prosthet. Dent.* **30**, 745-8.
Ireland E.J. (1983) Dental practice burnout. *Compend. Cont. Educ. Dent.* **4**, 367-9.
Jackson E. (1975) Establishing rapport. 1. Verbal interaction. *J. Oral Med.* **30**, 105-10.

Jackson E. (1978a) Patients' perceptions of dentistry. In *Advances in Behavioral Research in Dentistry* (Weinstein P., ed.). Seattle, Washington: University of Washington, Dept. of Community Dentistry.

Jackson E. (1978b) Convergent evidence for the effectiveness of interpersonal skill training for dental students. *J. Dent. Educ.* **42**, 517–23.

Jenny J., Frazier P. J., Bagramian R. A. et al. (1973) Parents' satisfaction and dissatisfaction with their children's dentist. *J. Public Health Dent.* **33**, 211–21.

Kent G. (1984) Satisfaction with dental care. *Medical Care* **22**, 583–5.

Kent G. (1987) Stress amongst dentists. In *Stress in Health Professionals* (Payne R., Firth-Cozens J., eds). Chichester: Wiley.

Kent G., Clarke P., Dalrymple-Smith D. (1981) The patient is the expert. *Med. Educ.* **15**, 38–42.

Kreisberg L., Treiman B. R. (1962) Dentists and the practice of dentistry as viewed by the public. *J. Am. Dent. Assoc.* **64**, 806–21.

Lefer L., Pleasure M. A., Rosenthal L. A. (1962) A psychiatric approach to the denture patient. *Psychosom. Res.* **6**, 199–207.

Levy R. L., Domoto P. K., Olson D. G. et al. (1980) Evaluation of one-to-one behavioural training. *J. Dent. Educ.* **44**, 221–2.

Locker D., Burman D., Otchere D. (1989) Work-related stress and its predictors among Canadian dental assistants. *Community Dent. Oral Epidemiol.* **17**, 263–6.

Ludwick W.E., Schnoebelen E.O., Knowdler D. (1964) *Greater Utilisation of Dental Technicians. II. Report of Clinical Tests.* Mimeograph. Great Lakes, Illinois: US Naval Training Center, Dental Research Facility.

Maguire P., Rutter D. (1976) Teaching medical students to communicate. In *Communication between Doctors and Patients* (Bennett A. E. ed.,). Oxford: Oxford University Press.

McKeithen E. J. (1966) The patient's image of the dentist. *J. Am. Coll. Dent.* **33**, 87–107.

Melamed B. G., Bennett C. G., Jerrell G. et al. (1983) Dentists' behavior management as it affects compliance and fear in pediatric patients. *J. Am. Dent. Assoc.* **196**, 324–30.

O'Shea R.M., Corah N., Ayer W. (1984) Sources of dentists' stress. *J. Am. Dent. Assoc.* **109**, 48–51.

Rankin J.A., Harris M. (1985) Patients' preferences for dentists' behaviors. *J. Am. Dent. Assoc.* **110**, 323–7.

Russek H. I. (1962) Emotional stress and coronary heart disease in American physicians, dentists and lawyers. *Am. J. Med. Sci.* **243**, 716–25.

Sachs R.H., Zullo T.G., Close J.M. (1981) Concerns of entering dental students. *J. Dent. Educ.* **45**, 133–6.

Schwartz R.M., Elgenbrode C., Contor O. (1984) A comprehensive stress reduction program for dental students. *J. Dent. Educ.* **48**, 203–7.

Skogedal O., Heloe L. A. (1979) Public opinions of dentists in Norway. *Community Dent. Oral Epidemiol.* **7**, 65–8.

Stacey D. C., Slome B. A., Musgrave D. (1978) Factors affecting patient completion of treatment in a student dental clinic. *J. Dent. Educ.* **42**, 609–17.

Stiles W. B., Putnam S. M., James S. A. et al. (1979) Dimensions of patient and physician roles in medical screening interviews. *Soc. Sci. Med.* **13A**, 335–41.

Szasz T. S., Hollender M. H. (1956) A contribution to the philosophy of medicine: the basic models of the doctor–patient relationship. *Arch. Intern. Med.* **97**, 585–92.

Tisdelle D.A., Hansen D., St. Lawrence J., Brown J. (1984) Stress management training for dental students. *J. Dent. Educ.* **48**, 196–201.

Vaillant G. E., Sobovale N. C., McArthur C. (1972) Some psychologic vulnerabilities of physicians. *N. Engl. J. Med.* **287**, 372–5.

Van Groenestijn M. A., Maas de Waal C. J., Mileman P. A. et al. (1980) The image of the dentist. *Soc. Sci. Med.* **14A**, 533–40.

Weinstein P., Nathan J. (1988) The challenge of fearful and phobic children. In *Dental Phobia and Anxiety. Dental Clinics of North America.* (Rubin J.G., Kaplan A., eds). London: Harcourt Brace Jovanovich.

Weinstein P., Getz T., Ratener P. et al. (1982) The effect of dentists' behaviors on fear-related behaviors in children. *J. Am. Dent. Assoc.* **104,** 32–8.

Weinstein P., Milgrom P., Ratener P. et al. (1979) Patient dental values and their relationship to oral health status, dentist perceptions and quality of care. *Community Dent. Oral Epidemiol.* **7,** 121–7.

Wills T. A. (1978) Perceptions of clients by professional helpers. *Psychol. Bull.* **85,** 968–1000.

Wurster C. A., Weinstein P., Cohen A. J. (1979) Communication patterns and pedodontics. *Percept. Mot. Skills* **48,** 159–66.

Young T.M. (1975) Questionnaire on the need for resuscitation in the dental surgery. *Anaesthesia* **30,** 391–401.

Appendix 1

Some help for students

Studying

Many students find studying difficult and this can be a source of stress and worry, especially when examinations are close at hand. The dental undergraduate course has a considerable number of degree and class examinations and it can sometimes be a problem to 'get down' to studying regularly. As a result the work can pile up and the amount of information to be learnt can appear overwhelming. This leads to feelings of anxiety which in turn make concentration difficult. A vicious circle can develop.

This situation is in many ways similar to the one that many irregular attenders find themselves in. Visiting the dentist might be put off for a variety of reasons. After a period, anxiety about the consequences of neglect begins (i.e. worries about what the dentist might find, or a concern about being criticized for not attending sooner), which makes the decision to attend that much harder. In such circumstances it may only be after symptoms begin to interfere with daily activities that an appointment is made. Similarly, students sometimes do not seek help with their work until the consequences of their neglect become serious, such as failing an exam. For patients and students loss of a tooth or loss of a year from dental school are consequences to be avoided if possible. If you find that the work is getting on top of you, an early visit to a lecturer or tutor may be less painful than you anticipate.

Some of the ideas discussed in Chapter 2 on prevention of dental ill health can be applied to preventing failure in examinations. In one research project, students were initially asked to monitor their own study methods, noting when and where they usually revised. They were encouraged to work in only one or two places which were not used for socializing. To increase motivation, the students were asked to do two things. First, to make a list of all the reasons why they should revise. Second, to reward themselves whenever they studied for a specified length of time. At first this time was short, about 20 min, but this increased as the programme progressed. They chose their own reinforcers, which could have been food, or watching television. Their studying time was plotted on a graph so they could see the results of their efforts. The programme was supplemented by information about how to revise. The results were very encouraging. A significant improvement in grades was found in the university examinations for these students compared with those who were not involved in the programme or who dropped out after the introduction. The essential point of this programme was to have the students select an easy task at first (20 min of studying) and then gradually increase this upwards over several weeks.

The method used to encourage accurate and efficient study was the SQ3R: survey, question, read, recite, review (Robinson, 1946).

Survey: Glance over the headings in the chapter to see the 3–6 main points. This survey should not take more than a minute. If the chapter has a final summary paragraph this will also list the main ideas. This survey will help you organize the ideas as you read them later.

Question: Now turn the first heading into a question. This will arouse your curiosity and bring to mind information you already know. The question will make the important points stand out as you read to find the answer.

Read: Read to answer that question by actively searching for information.

Recite: Having read the section, look away from the book and try to formulate the answer to your question. Use your own words and name an example. If you can do this, you know the material; if you can't, glance over the section again. A good way to do this is to jot down cue phrases in outline form on a sheet of paper. Make these notes very brief. Sometimes students believe that they have to know *everything*. You don't.

Now repeat steps 2, 3 and 4 for each section. That is, turn the next heading into a question, read to answer that question, and recite the answer by jotting down the cue phrases in your outline. Read in this way until the entire chapter is completed.

Review: When you have finished the chapter, look over your notes to get a bird's-eye view of the points and their relationship. Check your memory by covering up the notes and trying to recall the main points. Then expose each major point and try to recall the subpoints under it.

Anxiety during examinations

In Chapter 4, the use of cognitive modification in alleviating anxiety was discussed. This technique involves helping patients identify and modify the negative thoughts they repeat to themselves. Cognitive modification has also been found effective in helping students cope with examinations. Sitting an exam is in many ways similar to visiting a dentist, in that as the event approaches anxiety levels typically rise to a peak just before entering the examination hall. 'Test anxiety' refers to the anxiety some students feel when they are taking examinations. This can interfere with the ability to think clearly and perform well. It seems that many students with this difficulty dwell on self-deprecating thoughts and ruminate on the performance of others in the examination hall rather than concentrating on their own work. In other words, there seems to be a failure to attend to the relevant aspects of the task. Students have reported a preoccupation with such thoughts as 'I'll never get through this exam. Look at how well other people are working'.

In an attempt to help students with this problem, Meichenbaum (1972) encouraged them to become aware of their distracting thoughts during exams. They were then asked to imagine themselves in the examination hall but, instead of ruminating on irrelevant thoughts they were to instruct themselves positively. For example, to say to themselves: 'This is a difficult exam, I'd better start working on it' rather than: 'I'm really nervous. I can't handle this'. Compared to students waiting to take this programme, the procedure had a significant effect on both grades and self-reports of anxiety.

Conducting research projects

Some dental schools now ask their senior students to conduct a small research project as part of their degree. Often this can be a daunting prospect, but it needn't be. Research is a human enterprise, open to anyone who asks questions. Although many of the studies reported in this book have been done by 'professional researchers' who have financial support, some of the more interesting and helpful studies have been reported by individual dentists with a particular interest. A student or dental practitioner is in an excellent position to assess the effects of dental care or to assess changes of practice. An interest in research can lead not only to improvements in service but also a greater day-to-day interest and job satisfaction.

One of the more useful definitions of science is 'curiosity tempered by discipline'. We are all behavioural scientists in our daily lives, making predictions about what will occur in the future, trying things out, and noting the results. Being both excited and curious about a topic is necessary (if only to keep up motivation when the work is not going to plan), but so too is discipline. The only difference in a scientific undertaking is that it is important to be very clear about the objectives of the project, how they are tested, and the findings.

Hodgson and Rollnick (in Parry and Watts, see below) provide a useful introduction to planning research. They suggest that several features of doing research need to be kept in mind. They include the following:

1 Getting started will take at least as long as data collection.
2 The number of available subjects you can examine, question or observe will be one-10th of your first estimate.
3 Completion of a research project will take twice as long as your last estimate and three times as long as your first estimate.
4 A research project will change twice in the middle.
5 The help provided by other people has a half-life of two weeks.

Another important thing to remember about research is that there is no one 'right way' to do it. In the behavioural sciences, researchers have used formal questionnaires, individual interviews, group interviews, observations of behaviour, asking people to keep structured diaries of behaviour and feelings, analysing records and experiments, amongst others. The choice of method will depend on several factors, including time and other available resources, ethical considerations and intrusiveness as well as the nature of the question. A vital resource is the library: the *Index to the Dental Literature* and computer-based searches can provide invaluable help in accessing previous studies which help in formulating questions and choosing methods.

Further reading

Some books and articles that will help you are:

Bell J. (1987) *Doing your Research Project: A Guide for First-time Researchers in Education and Social Science.* Milton Keynes: Open University Press.
Brenner M., Brown J. and Canter D. (1985) *The Research Interview: Uses and Approaches.* London: Academic Press.
Meichenbaum D. (1972) Cognitive modification of test anxious college students. *J. Consult. Clin. Psychol.* **39**, 370–80.
Parry G. and Watts F. (1989) *Behavioural and Mental Health Research: A Handbook of Skills and Methods.* London: Erlbaum.
Sudman, S. and Bradburn N. (1982) *Asking Questions: A Practical Guide to Questionnaire Design.* San Francisco: Josy Bass.
Robinson, F. (1946) *Effective Study.* New York: Harper & Row.

Appendix 2

Case studies

The purpose of this appendix is to provide practice in applying some of the ideas and techinques outlined in the book. Four case studies are provided. After reading each one, consider how you might react to the situations portrayed.

Case study 1

The headteacher of the secondary school close to your practice comes to see you. She asks if you would give a dental health education talk to the early school-leavers (those leaving full-time education at 16). The school is in an area of high unemployment. How would you go about your task?

The first point to consider is whether the community dental service has a dental officer assigned to the school. If so, then it might be more appropriate if the community service undertook the talk. However it would be sensible to discuss the situation with the senior administrative dental officer. This person should have a clear idea of the major dental problems for adolescents in this area of the city. Given that the school is in a deprived area, these are usually poor plaque control, early periodontal disease and irregular dental attendance.

You will need to ensure that the headteacher has cleared your involvement with the education authority. Next you need to know how much time you have. Two or three short periods, rather than one long slot, will give you the opportunity to concentrate on one message at a time and to remind them of information given earlier. Authoritarian figures may alienate these adolescents. Dental health will be peripheral to many of their lifestyles and future health benefits may be of little concern, but dating and appearance are major interests. Early school-leavers are a difficult audience. A programme does not require visual aids but a supply of toothbrushes would be useful. It could involve:

Visit 1: Describe how the smile is an important part of appearance and sexuality and show that modern dentistry can save smiles painlessly. Discuss gum disease and how bad breath can be avoided.

Visit 2: For hygiene instruction and a practical demonstration of brushing, the class could be split into small groups. Using a science lesson may be a useful way to introduce the concept of plaque removal.

Visit 3: Evaluate the students' brushing skills through self-monitoring. After reiterating the importance of visiting the dentist, give out the names and addresses of local dentists who are keen to see young adults. Finally, an open discussion on dental problems might be useful.

Case study 2

Mrs A, aged 31, brings her 8-year-old daughter Susan to your office reporting that Susan has been complaining about a toothache for the past 2 weeks. Although the family has lived in the area for several years, they have not registered with a dentist previously. Mrs B has one other child, aged 3. The daughter is somewhat apprehensive but responds well to your guidance and explanations during the examination. You find that she has two rather deep lesions and you notice that Mrs A is visibly shaken when you say that Susan will require restorations. When you ask Mrs A about her own visiting pattern, she reports that she has not seen a dentist since she was a teenager. 'Now and then' she has 'twinges' from her teeth but these are 'no trouble at all'. How might you help this family and their future care?

It seems likely that Mrs A has been reluctant to visit a dentist on her child's behalf because of her own high level of anxiety. It is possible that she is feeling ashamed of her fears and her avoidance and may be expecting you to criticize her for neglecting her child's pain. Thus it is important to be non-judgemental in your approach and comments. Despite the lack of professional care Susan's oral health is reasonably good, so that Mrs A may be well motivated to take on any further preventive measures which may be appropriate.

There are two strands in helping this family. The first is to take particular care with the daughter. Since she does not seem to be unduly distressed, she could serve as a model for the mother. It may be worthwhile taking the risk of asking the mother to stay in the surgery, out of the daughter's line of sight, during the restorations. Your behaviour will be closely scrutinized. The second strand is to treat the mother gradually, over a number of sessions. There is a strong possibility that she will break an appointment made for herself unless she comes to believe that you are there to help rather than to judge.

Case study 3

Mr B, aged 75, keeps an appointment made by his eldest son for the replacement of his full (top and bottom) denture. Mr B states that he has come only because his son insisted. He says that he had difficulty in adapting to his present appliance when it was fitted 10 years ago. Although he has a great deal of trouble eating solid foods, he claims that he is managing sufficiently well and his diet is reasonable. Not being in the best of health, he does not expect to live much longer anyway. The effort would be 'wasted' on him. His appliance is quite dirty. What further information would you gather, and what possible steps could you take?

There are several important aspects of this presentation. The first is that you need to know much more about Mr B's family and current living conditions. Whether his spouse is still alive is crucial, but the proximity of children and the availability of other social supports are also important. Mr B's diet is relevant. The ways in which Mr B describes himself and his future, as well as the state of his appliance, may indicate that he has become depressed, a common problem in elderly people. Non-verbal cues are important here, especially a slumping posture and a lack of eye contact. Should it seem likely that Mr B is in emotional trouble, there is an ethical and professional obligation to ensure that there is some follow-up. Mr B's general medical practitioner could be asked to make a home visit.

There is also the question of whose needs would be met by a new appliance. On the one hand, Mr B may be hoping for some help with his denture but is reticent about asking, preferring instead to justify his need by quoting his son's concern. On the other hand, it may be the son's difficulty in accepting Mr B's right to adjust in his own way to increasing age which needs to be addressed. The task of the dentist here is to find the delicate balance between acknowledging Mr B's request to be left alone and intervening in an appropriate way.

Case study 4

You have had a long and busy day. Mr C arrives just a few minutes before you had planned to leave for a game of squash. He begins by complaining that he has been experiencing severe pain in his upper jaw for the past week, since you performed a restoration on a molar. You remember that you were in a hurry that day and felt a little unhappy about your work. Mr C demands that you do something about it immediately since he does not have the time to come back during the next week. The dental hygienist states that she is fed up of working late without notice and will not stay on today because of a commitment. You lose your temper. The hygienist leaves, threatening to quit; the patient says that he will tell his friends about your incompetence and, to make matters worse, you lose your squash game. That evening you brood on this incident, running it over in your mind many times and chastising yourself. Are there any ways to prevent a similar situation developing in the future?

It may seem that the best way to prevent such an incident is to be certain that every piece of work is perfect, so there would never be any grounds for complaint. This is clearly unrealistic. Everyone involved in this situation is under stress. Although the dentist may have left the amalgam a little high on the patient's last visit, this may be important only because Mr C is in the habit of clenching his teeth as a reaction to stress. The hygienist may be feeling taken for granted, as well as underpaid. The dentist seems to be working very hard, requires very high standards, and may find it difficult to express personal difficulties.

Some reconsideration of office management and personal views about work is needed. Most large and successful businesses invest time and energy in personnel development, often by hiring a consultant to examine working practices and staff relationships. In this case, a consultant may recommend that the dental team attend a day's workshop so that problems and feelings can be aired. Although expensive, so too is the cost of training new staff. It would also be helpful for the dentist to examine his or her beliefs about working practices. The anger may have been a result of some erroneous assumptions such as 'My efforts should be appreciated by all my patients and staff' or 'I should be thoroughly competent and successful in everything I do'.

Index

bis after a reference number indicates that a topic is separately mentioned on the same page of the text: *passim* indicates that the references are scattered throughout the pages mentioned.

Accurate empathy, 150–3
Analgesia (*see also* Pain, Placebo effect)
  effects of, 99, 100, 106
  general, 78, 91, 154–5
  hypnotic, 114–6
  local, 77, 110, 135
  predicting need for, 108, 117
  relative, 78–9
  requests for, 108, 7
Antecedents to preventive care, 33, 34
Anxiety,
  aetiology of, 66–74, 77
  and behaviour, 56, 63–6, 69, 151
  in children, 63–73 *passim*, 77–89 *passim*, 145–6, 149
  and classical conditioning, 71–2, 73
  definition, 56
  and disruption, 1–2, 145–6
  and fear, 56
  measurement of, 58–66, 146
  and pain, 66–7, 77, 101, 109, 135
  and personality, 55–6, 85–6
  reduction of, 77–96, 145–6, 149, 166
    choosing between therapies, 94–5
    clinical psychology, 95
    cognitive, 62, 92–4
    control, 87, 93
    emotional support, 87–9, 94, 135–6,
    hypnosis, 114–7
    information, 82–6
    modelling, 80–82
    patients' advice, 95
    pharmacological, 78–9
    relaxation, 82–92
  self-reports of, 56, 58, 62
  state, 58–9, 90
  in students, 162–3
  trait, 58–9

Anxiety (*cont.*)
  and type of dental procedure, 56–8, 61, 81, 87, 91–2, 151
  and visiting patterns, 14, 55, 56, 58, 65, 69, 73, 166
Appearance, 15, 22, 43, 51, 123–4, 165
Appointment keeping,
  and anxiety, 55, 66, 83, 166
  and satisfaction with care, 140–1, 153–4
Attendance (*see* Utilization)
Attitudes
  in dental students, 18, 141–2
Audio-analgesia, 112
Authoritarianism, 143–5

Barriers, to care, 14,
Behaviour,
  and anxiety, 56, 63–6, 151
  charting of, 39–40, 48
  non-verbal, 106–7, 146–9
  and pain, 106–9
  verbal, 145–6, 149–53
Beliefs (*see also* Attitudes, Health Belief Model)
  lay and professional, 21–3, 6–7, 13, 15–17, 125, 131–2, 138–9
Biofeedback, 89
Bruxism, 127

Capitation, 19–20
Caries, 4, 10–12, 19, 24, 31, 35
Charting, 39–40, 48
Classical conditioning, 71–2, 73, 102
Clinical psychologists, 95
Cognitive modification,
  and anxiety, 92–4, 113
  and pain, 112–3, 117–8
Competence, assessment of, 64, 136–40

Index

Compliance (*see* Prevention; Utilization)
Contracting, 51
Control, over dentist's behaviour, 87, 93, 113, 118
Counselling, 128

Dental Anxiety Scale, 59–60, 61, 66 *bis*
Dental procedures (*see also* Extractions; Injections; Restorations)
　and anxiety, 56–8, 61, 81, 87, 91–2, 151
　and pain, 66–7, 101, 103, 105–6
Dental students, 40–2, 57–8, 131, 143–56 *passim*,
　and test anxiety, 162–3, 155
　socialization of, 18, 155
Dental team, 33, 154, 156, 167–8
Dentists (*see also* Dentist–patient relationship)
　competence, 64, 136–40
　effect on patients' anxiety, 62, 70–1, 135–8, 145–6, 149
　effect on patients' pain, 135–6
　patients' selection of, 14, 136–42
　personality, 71, 135–8, 143–4
　stress in, 1–2, 55, 154–6
　views of dental procedures, 57–8, 142–3
　views of patients, 141–2
　views of patient's anxiety, 61, 66, 148
　views of patient's pain, 99
Dentist–patient relationship (*see also* Dentists; Treatment decisions)
　and communication, 142–54, 24
　and cooperative behaviour, 34, 114, 145–6, 149
　and patients' anxiety, 71, 82–9, 135–6
　and patients' view of dentistry, 22, 136–42
　and placebo effect, 135
　and stress in dentistry, 1–2, 154–6, 167–8
Dentures, 13, 37–42, 142–4, 166
Depression, 104, 127, 128, 167
Diet (*see also* Caries) 10–12, 19, 23, 35, 45, 47–9, 50
Disability, 5, 17, 125
Distraction, and anxiety, 92–3, 95
　and pain, 112–3,
'Draw-a-person' test, 84

Edentulism (*see also* Dentures) 5, 6, 8–9, 13, 21, 23, 24, 58, 129–30
Educational programmes (*see also* Prevention)
　and anxiety, 43–5
　effects of, 29–33, 37–8, 42–5, 165
　and personality, 45–7
Elderly (*see also* Dentures; Edentulism), 13, 14, 122, 129–30, 166
Emotional support, 87–9, 135
Epidemiology, 7–12, 24
Ethics, 4, 17, 18, 20–1, 122, 131, 167
Ethnic differences, 12

Extractions, as cause of anxiety, 56–8, 66–7, 69, 84–5, 86, 135–6
　as negative reinforcement, 42
　and pain, 106, 135–6
Eye gaze, 147–8
Eysenck Personality Inventory, 72–3, 108

Fear (*see* Anxiety)
Feedback, to dentist, 153–4
Flossing, consequences of, 35
　in educational programmes, 30–1
Fluoridation, 12, 19, 23, 29, 37–8, 77

Gate Theory, 100–3, 105, 109, 113–4
Gestures, 148

Handicap, 5, 16, 17, 122, 130–2
Health, definition of, 4–8
Health Belief Model, 15, 37
Hypnosis, 79, 114–7, 127

Iatrogenic illness, 23
Impairment, 5, 122
Injections, and anxiety, 56–8, 72, 87
　and pain, 100 *bis*, 101, 135–6
Immunity, 122 *bis*, 126

Locus of control, 45–7, 86

McGill Pain Questionnaire, 105–6
Memory, 32, 69
Mental handicap, 49–50, 130–2
Modelling, 40–2
　and anxiety, 70, 82
　and preventive care, 40–2
　and socialization, 40, 149

Neuroticism (*see* Eysenck Personality Inventory)
Norms, 3–4, 14–5
Non-verbal communication, 106, 146–9, 167

Oral health (*see* Flossing; Toothbrushing; Prevention)
Orthodontics, 21–2, 123–5, 155

Pain
　and anxiety, 66–7, 77, 99, 101, 109, 135–6
　chronic vs acute, 103–4
　clinical vs induced, 103
　and dental procedures, 5, 56–8, 66–7, 101,
　emotional component, 101, 105, 111–3
　evaluative component, 101, 105, 113–8
　expectations of, 55, 66–7, 101 *bis*, 114, 117–4
　experience of, 5, 13, 67, 68–9, 72, 99–104
　and injury, 99–102
　and phobias, 69, 109
　placebo effect, 110–1

Pain (*cont.*)
  reduction of, 109–18
    psychological, 110–8
    pharmacological, 103, 106, 109–11
  sensory component, 101, 105, 109–11
  somatogenic vs psychogenic, 102
  of temporomandibular joint, 6, 13, 22, 104, 125–9
  thresholds, 67, 72, 103, 109
  tolerance, 67, 72, 103
  of toothache, 105, 106
Parents, effects on child's anxiety, 69–70, 81, 83–4, 89
  involvement in child's care, 4, 22, 39–40, 51, 123, 131–2, 151
  presence in surgery, 81, 89, 151
  views of dental care, 4, 11, 22, 137–8
Performance Gap, 19
Personal space, 148
Personality
  and anxiety, 72–3, 85–6
  and cooperation, 123
  of dentist, 70–1, 135–9 *passim*, 143–5
  and pain, 105, 125–6
  and prevention, 45–7
Periodontal disease, 4, 5, 8, 19 *bis*, 42, 131, 165
Phobias (*see also* Anxiety; Pain), 56, 57–8, 69, 73, 81, 109
Physical environment, 138–9, 146–7
Physiological arousal, 72–3
  and pain, 68, 100, 104, 107
  as correlate of anxiety, 89–92
  as measure of anxiety, 56–9, 61, 62–3, 89–91
Placebo effect, 91, 110–1, 135–6
Plaque, consequences of, 35
  and disclosing agents, 30–1, 42–3
  meaning of, 33
  and personality, 45–7
  reduction of, 37–47 *passim*, 50, 165
Posture, 148
Preparedness, 67
Prevention (*see also* Dentist–patient relationship; Educational programmes; Reinforcement; Utilization)
  and appearance, 43–51, 165
  and beliefs, 10–12, 14–5, 37–8, 42, 43–51
  and cost, 14
  design of a preventive programme, 19, 47–52
  and education, 9, 29–33, 42
  and handicap, 49–50, 122, 131
  and modelling, 40–2
  and personality, 45–7
  and satisfaction, 140
  and stress in dentists, 2
  vs treatment, 19, 20–4
Proximity, 148–9
Psychology, definition, 2–3
Punishment, 4, 34, 45, 82

Quality of life, 6–7, 15–16, 108–9

Reading ease, 32–3
Reinforcement (*see also* Prevention; Punishment)
  and dentist's behaviour, 34, 153
  and modelling, 40–2, 81
  negative, 34, 42
  positive, 34, 36–42
  and preventive care, 34–52
  selection of, 36, 38, 40, 51 *bis*
  self-reinforcement, 40, 51 *bis*
  and shaping, 49–50
  for studying, 161–2
  vs education, 37–8
Relative analgesia, 78–9
Relaxation
  and anxiety, 89–92
  by biofeedback, 89
  by hypnosis, 79, 114–7
  by muscle relaxation, 90, 93, 126–7
  and pain, 109
  and systematic desensitization, 91–2
Research projects, 163–4
Research design,
  baseline measure, 48
  blind assessment, 39
  control groups, 30, 41–2, 91, 114
  cross-sectional vs longitudinal, 18
  interobserver agreement, 6, 64
  prospective vs retrospective, 15
  random assignment, 30
  self-reports, 9
  time-sampling, 64
Restorations, and anxiety, 56–8, 81, 166
  and pain, 113
  quality of, 19–20, 23, 64, 137–9, 142
Role, 5, 153

Satisfaction with care, 136–41 *passim*
Sex differences, 93, 108
Shaping, 49–50
Sickness Impact Profile, 6, 109
Social class, 7, 10–12, 137–8, 141
Social skills, 136–41, 149–54
Socialization, 4, 18, 149
Socio-economic level, and quality of care, 141–2
  and utilization, 4, 7, 10–1, 22
Sociology, definition of, 2–3
State–Trait Anxiety Inventory, 58–9, 61, 90–1
Studying, 161–2
Systematic desensitization, 91–2
Stereotypes, 129, 131–2, 141–2
Stress, 126–7, 154–7, 167–8
  management of, 127, 156, 168

Target behaviour, 49
Technical skill, and choice of dentist, 136–41 *passim*

Tell-Show-Do, 82–3
Temporomandibular joint disorder, 6, 13, 22, 104, 125–9
Thumbsucking, 39–40
Tooth shock, 103
Toothbrushing (*see also* Prevention; Reinforcement)
  in children, 30–1, 36, 50
  and mentally handicapped people, 49, 131
  norms about, 4, 166
  and shaping, 49–50
Touching, 148–9
Tranquillizers, 79
Treatment decisions, 19–24, 106, 123–5, 129, 142–5

Uncertainty (*see also* Anxiety)
  as cause of anxiety, 56, 68, 74
  reduction of, 82–7, 117–8

Utilization
  and accessibility, 9, 11, 14, 136, 147
  and age, 13, 14, 129
  and anxiety, 55–61 *passim*, 65, 73, 69
  and beliefs, 5, 10–12, 15–16
  choice of dentist, 136–41
  and consequences, 19, 22
  and cost, 9, 10, 14, 141–2
  demand vs need, 13–17
  and family, 16, 123–5
  and pain, 13, 19, 99
  and satisfaction with care, 140–1
  and social class, 8–17 *passim*, 22, 141, 165

Values, 3, 10, 18, 22
Verbal communication (*see* Dentist–patient relationship)
Vision (*see* Eye gaze)
Visual Analogue Scale, 104–5, 128

Work of worrying, 118

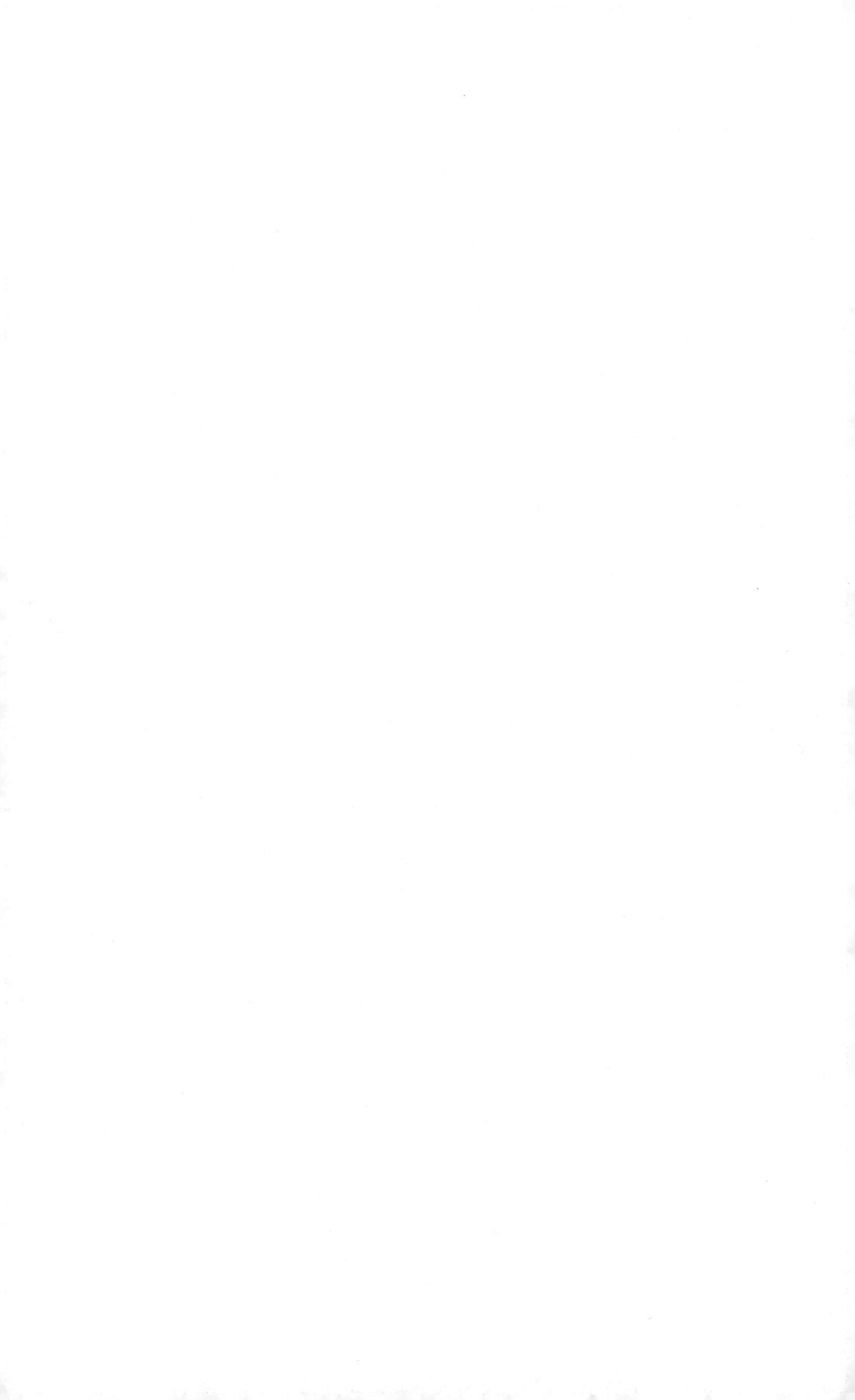